# FiNDing Hope

# FINDING HOPE

## The Mind-Body Connection and the Importance of Being Seen and Heard

### Jocelyn Bystrom

**Stone Tiger Books**

Copyright © 2023 Jocelyn Bystrom

First published by Stone Tiger Books in 2023.

All rights reserved; no part of this publication may be reproduced, stored in a retrieval system, or transmitted in any form or by any means, electronic, mechanical, photocopying, recording, or otherwise without the prior written permission of the Publisher. This book may not be lent, resold, hired out or otherwise disposed of by way of trade in any form of binding or cover other than that in which it is published, without the prior written consent of the Publisher.

ISBN: 9798989250103
eISBN: 9798989250110

Cover and Jacket design by Rob Carter

Stone Tiger Books
225 E. 35th Street, Ground Floor
New York, NY 10016
USA

Printed in the United States of America

*For Dale, my everything.
Infinite gratitude.*

*For Faith, that made Hope possible.*

*For Love, that connected & rooted.*

*For Family, who sheltered & lifted me with compassion.*

*For my team of trusted medical practitioners, thank you.*

*For Mom, who prioritized her girls; and went without.
For sowing seeds of faith, and a lifetime
of care. I love you, mama.*

# CONTENTS

Title Page
Copyright
Dedication
Introduction
PART ONE                                               1
I Dig                                                  3
Chapter One                                            5
Chapter Two                                           11
Chapter Three                                         17
Chapter Four                                          23
Chapter Five                                          29
Chapter Six                                           45
PART TWO                                              59
Chapter Seven                                         61
Chapter Eight                                         67
Chapter Nine                                          75
Chapter Ten                                           87
PART THREE                                            97
Chapter Eleven                                        99
Chapter Twelve                                       107
Chapter Thirteen                                     121

| | |
|---|---|
| Chapter Fourteen | 135 |
| Chapter Fifteen | 147 |
| Chapter Sixteen | 169 |
| Chapter Seventeen | 195 |
| Chapter Eighteen | 207 |
| Chapter Nineteen | 225 |
| PART FOUR | 239 |
| Chapter Twenty | 241 |
| Chapter Twenty-One | 245 |
| Chapter Twenty-Two | 269 |
| Chapter Twenty-Three | 287 |
| PART FIVE | 303 |
| Chapter Twenty-Four | 305 |
| Chapter Twenty-Five | 321 |
| Chapter Twenty-Six | 329 |
| Epilogue | 341 |
| References | 343 |
| Acknowledgement | 347 |
| About The Author | 355 |

# INTRODUCTION

> *There are losses that rearrange the world.... Pain that transports you to an entirely different universe, even while everyone else thinks nothing has really changed.*
>
> —MEGAN DEVINE, IT'S OK THAT YOU'RE NOT OK

*F*iNDing Hope is the story of a seven-year struggle against a rare but growing, and largely undiagnosed, mental health condition known as functional neurological disorder (FND) that left me with daily epileptic-like seizures, thunderous headaches, and the inability to work, drive, or care properly for myself or my family. Numerous hospital admissions concluded without a clear diagnosis, and a palpable fear of death prevailed as I experienced severe cognitive and physical decline.

Despite doctors' best efforts, and in a world where, according to Johns Hopkins Medicine in 2022, "an estimated 26 percent of Americans ages eighteen and older—one in four adults—suffers from a diagnosable mental health disorder in any given year," millions of people worldwide may be struggling with undiagnosed FND. In this work, *The Myth of Normal*, leading trauma expert Dr. Gabor Mate observes that the current medical paradigm "reduces complex events to their biology, and it separates mind from body, concerning itself almost exclusively with one or the other without appreciating their essential unity." *FiNDing Hope* highlights this critical need for "essential unity" as I navigated a medical system focused on biology rather than the essential mind-body connection.

Emerging experts who focus on this disorder—one that in past generations may have been dismissed as "hysteria" or even treated by exorcists—estimate that the prevalence of FND may be more common than epilepsy. However, with treatments based on a proper diagnosis, new research indicates that 60 percent of individuals with FND will experience improved symptoms—as I did.

FND complicates the nervous system, interfering with the normal pathways by which the brain and body sends and receives messages. It includes a variety of physical symptoms, which, for me, manifested in numerous, terrifying seizures, chronic pain, balance problems, migraine headaches, involuntary movements, sleep disturbances, and difficulties breathing, among other ailments. The disorder itself is triggered in diverse ways, including acute psychological trauma, physical injuries, and brain changes affected by other underlying physical or mental disorders. For me, it was the sudden and egregious loss of a job I loved and excelled at that led to a years-long cascade of debilitating health challenges.

But that was just the tip of the proverbial iceberg—the roots of my FND onset ultimately sank deep into the soil of my childhood.

*FiNDing Hope* is my unique experience of living with functional neurological disorder (FND) and learning to prioritize self-compassion and whole-body health, a journey that led me to recognize that caring for my health included caring for my physical, cognitive, mental, spiritual, and relational health.

Clinicians and experts, like Dr. Mate, explain trauma's origin and core as "a web of circumstances, relationships, events, and experiences." Or, in the words of Dr. Bessel van der Kolk in his foreword to *Trauma and Memory*, by Peter Levine: "Health and illness are not random states in a particular body or body part. They are, in fact, an expression of an entire life lived, one that cannot, in turn, be understood in isolation: it is influenced by—or better yet, it arises from—a web of circumstances, relationships, events, and experiences." He further summarizes trauma as "when we're not seen and known."

My book is structured to reflect a five-season narrative framework. Each "season" develops a particular theme that drives the story towards diagnostic clarity and a roadmap for wellness: trauma, reflection, waiting, clarity, and renewal. Readers are invited to sit beside me in the front seat of the world's tallest, longest, and fastest rollercoaster: that's what FND produces.

If we are to believe scientific studies by medical researchers studying the latest collected data in medicine and particularly neurology, why have most of us never heard of FND? Available medical research from the UK reports that between 50,000–100,000 individuals in 2020, in that country alone, were determined to be suffering from FND. How many of those, like me, grew increasingly more discouraged as they waited for a diagnosis? Based on the findings in the UK, it's likely that almost 13 million people globally experienced functional symptoms today, with or without a diagnosis. It's perplexing to imagine why neither the United States nor Canada have publicly available statistics about the prevalence of FND.

If our numbers are like those reported in the UK, by population, approximately 560,000 Americans and 63,000 Canadians may be experiencing functional symptoms or have an FND diagnosis. It took seven years and eleven specialists for me to receive an FND diagnosis. How much money is wasted nationally each year on neurological investigations only to learn that it's FND? Notably, the illness itself is not yet even listed on NAMI's or CMHA's lists of mental health conditions.

*FiNDing Hope* isn't a story of a miracle cure, or of recovery, after an FND diagnosis. More importantly, it's about the need for life-giving collaborative care that supports whole-body wellness, and our need for hope when any aspect of our health is jeopardized. I was willing to fight to get my joy-filled life back and needed help to accomplish it. There's no pill or a cure for FND, but hope abounds in every thread of the narrative fabric of this story.

# PART ONE

## SEASON OF TRAUMA

JOCELYN BYSTROM

# I DIG

*June 17, 2021*

I dig. No one watches. I'm alone. Sweat drips into my eyes, off my cheeks, and dampens my shirt. Tension cries out from taut, straining muscles. My back is tender from repetitive lifting. It's not easy digging here in my yard. The earth is full of rock, football-sized boulders wedged and embedded in clay. My only tools are a shovel and a mattock, which I've brought, knowing what lies beneath.

Finally, my task is complete. I kneel, looking around tentatively, appreciative that no other bears witness. My face and arms are covered with smudged sweat, tears leak down my face, and there's dirt embedded under my fingernails. Beyond beat, I reach out and grasp the envelope from where it lies, on the other side of the hole. With relief, I hold the letter, knowing it will soon be buried.

I pick up the lighter I brought along and flick the switch. I'm mesmerized as I watch the paper's slow burn. Ash glides effortlessly like a gull on the sea breeze, then falls with gravity into the newly excavated grave. I reach across to where I've piled earth, fingers seeking. I collect and sprinkle soil atop the ashes, and continue to do so till they are covered, extinguished, buried.

JOCELYNBYSTROM

# CHAPTER ONE

### What's the Emergency?

*January 23, 2021*

"Nine one one. What's your emergency?"

"There's a lady here," the clerk replied. "Her husband says she's having a seizure. In our store."

This was not my first, second, or even tenth seizure. Not even my first that day. There'd been another that morning — a whopper, more than twenty minutes.

Anxious thoughts infiltrated as I remembered it.

Exhausted, I had nodded off in the recliner. I experienced central apnea and my brain forgot to tell my body to breathe, and it began. My head shook gently back and forth, as if I were saying no., I tried to snap the fingers of my left hand, our prearranged seizure signal. My right hand, usually rigid as a seizure begins, had become a claw.

Dale had been enjoying his relaxed Saturday morning, reading the news on his iPad while sipping Earl Grey tea. But when the seizure took over, he knew. There was crashing and banging, and he grabbed his phone as he rushed over to me. He dialed 911.

Paramedics arrived just as the seizure ended.

Breathless, I was on the floor in the recovery position. The now empty recliner had been wounded in battle — its mechanism couldn't withstand the violence as I seized. A short while later, Dale told my neurologist that the event lasted twenty-two minutes.

After lunch, to take our minds off the earlier chaos, Dale suggested we go for a drive. A great idea, I thought. I hadn't been able to drive for almost a year, and often felt desperate to regain my license and my ability to freely grab car keys and go.

~

January 27, a year earlier in 2020, had become a date forever etched in my memory. That day, my neurologist first made strict recommendations as precautionary measures regarding my condition. I'd stood in my bedroom, after leaving the noisy family room to ensure privacy, and was told, "No driving or employment, effective immediately."

An electroencephalogram three days earlier revealed "abnormal epileptiform discharges" had been discovered. I was at risk for an epileptic event. After the shock of not being able to return to work as an educator, the most impactful news was that I could no longer drive. My independence was stripped away without warning. Tears formed. I had recently returned to work in a new role as a teacher-librarian. It was work that I enjoyed immensely. I'd been back to work for only five months after my last medical leave and career retraining.

Ever so slowly, I'd walked back through our open plan, single great room that combines living, kitchen and dining areas with a central island, wondering how to tell my husband, Dale, without my mother overhearing. She was in a fragile state — newly diagnosed with dementia — and we'd planted seeds of having her move in with us.

As I told Dale my news, Mom spoke up (there was nothing wrong with her hearing). "Don't worry, dear," she said, "I can drive you anywhere you need to go."

"Thanks, Mom," I responded. Her offer, it turned out, hadn't been helpful. Two days later she likewise would lose her driver's license.

Through the fall of 2020, I experienced several small

seizures. But the first complex seizure of significant length and intensity arrived January 3, 2021. Another came the very next day. This would be the start of a fierce new escalating pattern.

Dale ordered me a Life Alert button mechanism to wear around my neck. I believe that he did this to slow *his* pounding heart.

~

So, after the morning seizure on January 23, 2021, had shattered our calm, we headed out for a drive on a sunny Saturday afternoon. Dale stopped briefly on the picturesque Dyke Road beside the K'ómoks estuary; he wanted to take a photograph, because of how splendid the ice-capped glacier had appeared the morning before on his way to work. We got out of the car and gazed up at the glacier. It was lovely to be embraced by the unexpected January warmth.

Soon we were back in the car. Dale is a romantic, and after thirty-eight years of marriage still consistently surprised me with first-date-like anticipation of where he was taking us. The sun glistened on the snow-peaked mountains. We drove south beside the sea, from the Comox Valley after leaving Courtenay. We stopped once more to walk, soak up the sound of the waves lapping on the shore, and breathed in the scent of drying algae that wafted up with the morning tide.

At Buckley Bay, we parked and walked hand in hand down a flight of stairs. We wanted to investigate a small sign that we'd seen before but hadn't checked out. It read, *More Shops This Way.* We popped into Fanny Bay Oysters, a seafood shop where we'd occasionally go to buy oysters, clams, and our favourite, candied salmon. Then we moved on to explore shops that were new to us.

"How are you doing?" Dale asked. "Do you want to go in?"

I was feeling light-headed. But I agreed we should look in the eclectic little gift shop in front of us. Dale led the way while I held his arm for support. On display was an interesting variety of items, including fruits and vegetables, fresh-baked bread, locally made sauces, and handcrafted art from regional and indigenous artists. By the cashier, I saw Denman Island's famous chocolate, cleverly placed to seduce tourists in a holiday mood while they waited for the ferry.

And then this happened.

My breathing suddenly shallowed. My head began to sway. Dale was in front of me, and I reached out and grasped him — first his arm, then his body.

"It's happe—" escaped my mouth, but I couldn't finish.

Panicked voices surrounded me, but I couldn't see whose. Wide-eyed, I sought my husband.

My voice had been silenced. I was in a tiny hidden gem of a gift shop, and my mind cried, *Get me out of here.*

Dale instantly recognized what was happening. As the seizure took control, Dale held me. "My wife is having a problem," he said to a clerk. "Do you have a chair? And call nine one one—she's having a seizure."

He guided me gently, and I felt something bump the back of my legs. I sat.

The clerk was talking to a 911 dispatcher: "It's still happening. She's seated. Her husband—he's holding her."

My arms and legs thrashed. Each time one movement stopped, and I prayed it would end, another started. I was terrified. My head jerked back and forth. *Help! I don't want to knock works of art off shelves. Get me out of here.* Again, I tried to communicate with my eyes and failed.

I heard sirens approaching for the second time that day. It was my first seizure in public, and I was embarrassed to be causing such a fuss. Then my head crashed back into the glass countertop of the cashier's desk. I felt Dale's gentle hands protecting my brain from colliding with the counter again.

I heard the clerk tell the 911 operator that the paramedics had arrived.

I was still seizing. The stretcher didn't fit through the door into the shop. It was that confined. After some maneuvering, I was outside, and my body collapsed as if I'd run a marathon. My thoughts raced to cross the line and comprehend.

I don't have epilepsy — my neurology team had been clear on that — and unlike most epileptics I'm fully conscious throughout my seizures. Lids glued shut at the climax of the seizure, opened to surrounding chaos, seeking my love. The paramedics were covering, buckling, and restraining me. Darting pupils methodically located Dale after homing in on their target. He appeared relieved. I was in expert hands. His eyes delivered a sought-after message and regulated mine.

We were off. The ambulance headed to Courtenay and the North Island Hospital's emergency department from Buckley Bay. Until I sensed my breaths slow. I couldn't get enough air in my lungs. My body began to seize again and the strap restraining me for my protection edged higher. It was now across my throat. I stopped breathing.

JOCELYN BYSTROM

# CHAPTER TWO

### What Is Trauma?

Trauma isn't what happened to me, it's what happened inside me *because of* what happened. It's both an open and invisible wound simultaneously. I wasn't always aware of this.

By the age of ten, I thought traumatic incidents happened to others—to soldiers, firefighters, and people in third world countries. At seventeen, I read news stories and viewed unsettling images only if I happened to have watched the six o'clock news. Years later, on September 11, 2001, at 8:45 a.m., I was glued to our thirty-seven-inch television screen, witnessing the live coverage of 9/11. Mesmerized, I knelt in horror as terrorized individuals leapt to their deaths, rather than burn in the flames when militants hijacked airplanes and carried out four coordinated terror attacks. *That*, I believed, was capital "T" trauma.

Catastrophic natural disasters were transmitted to previously naïve ears. And when later I learned about horrific abuse toward indigenous children in Canada's residential schools, I counted my blessings. I'd been changed by knowledge of war and abuse. Trauma, occurred in the trenches, and to mothers who lost sons in battle, so that I could enjoy freedom. I taught seventh and eighth grade history in 2005 and learned alongside my students about the more insidious aftermath and enduring effects of war. These were what came to mind when I questioned and responded to the query, "What is trauma?"

I was knowledgeable in 2013, about the effects of post-traumatic stress and the repercussions of traumatic incidents on my students and students' behaviour. Behaviours which expressed secrets, lies and betrayals, and affected my students' ability to learn. Innocent lives changed by circumstances, over which they held no control. I taught students who'd suffered from poverty, abuse, abandonment, and neglect. And those who experienced a death of their sense of safety.

What I hadn't known at fifty was that trauma leaves its mark on both the mind and body.

~

I began having what the doctor later called atypical "spells" involving forward flexion in the spring of 2013. A prescribed medication trial aimed to reduce them instead triggered side effects. Medication was met with resistance as my body fought for control.

My doctor, a general practitioner (GP), suggested an additional diagnosis of generalized anxiety disorder (GAD) and prescribed a second medication which also caused immediate and frightening side effects. The medications made me feel like I was losing control of my mind and caused severe migraines. These medication trials left me fearful and reinforced a childhood strategy and impulse for greater self-discipline.

*Don't let others steal your joy or take custody of your mind*, became my unspoken mantra. As a child and young adult, I managed circumstances within my control and mastered the masks of poise and calm. No one would learn that I was in fact an imposter. Appearances mattered, and I jealously guarded my heart and narrowed who I'd trust.

Anger percolated.

I never experienced any desire to experiment with drugs or alcohol as a teen. I was an outlier, a year younger than my peers, and consciously flew under the radar. Inconspicuous was the safer choice. I hadn't wanted to feel powerless. I despised that feeling. It was my experience of childhood and left me uncertain and filled with fear.

Why, I wondered in the spring of 2013, was my body so resistant to medication? Prescribed pharmaceuticals were withdrawn and ruled out as possible factors that caused atypical movements.

Only one thing seemed helpful to slow the increasing reoccurrence of what were now unexpected body jerks. I'd squeeze every muscle throughout my core and legs, like an oyster using its adductor muscle to keep its shell closed. With every muscle taut, I could stand without assistance for short periods. But holding this level of tension in my body throughout my workday as a teacher left me exhausted by mid-morning.

At the suggestion of a keen locum, who'd filled in while my family doctor was away on summer holidays, I began a new season of medical investigation, which turned out to be the beginning of a seven-year season of waiting and wondering, meeting with specialists, and more waiting.

Why, I continued to wonder, was I experiencing these strange physical phenomena? Why me? And why now? I waited between appointments with a heavy heart and increasing uncertainty.

In November 2013, I had my first EEG, requested by the locum. He'd been curious, as I was. A passionate, newly trained young professional, like I'd been at twenty-four as a first-year teacher. We both hoped to discover why I was experiencing unexpected jerks, and I don't mean the annoying jerks who make every conversation about themselves and who are habitually late and not respectful of anyone's time.

That first EEG showed that there were indeed abnormalities. They discovered generalized spike and wave discharges suggestive of one of the rarer epilepsy syndromes. There was a hint of, but no formal diagnosis. A follow-up EEG with sleep deprivation was requested by the neurologist who'd read my initial EEG test results. An EEG, I learned, detects electrical activity in the brain as brain cells communicate via electrical impulses, even when we sleep.

*Did I have epilepsy*? I investigated to satiate my curiosity and increasing concern as new possible diagnoses were bantered back and forth by specialists. I completed preliminary research online after one neurologist hinted, that I had it.

I was surprised to learn that the type of discharge they'd noted was more common in adolescents. I was in my late forties at the time. Curiosity prompted additional exploring. I read bits and bytes about the history of epilepsy and discovered many of what my daughter called "fun facts." We're kinda science geeks, and delight in knowledge acquired through study, experience or being taught. I learned that it was William Spartling, who first used the term "epileptologist" for a physician specializing in epilepsy at the beginning of the twentieth century.

I was shocked to learn that epilepsy and seizures are very common. One in twelve people will experience a seizure during their lifetime. *Really?* I questioned. Most of the so-called facts would need to be verified for accuracy before I believed them. I searched various academic websites for details to confirm, validate, or dismiss untruths. I am inherently distrustful and wary of content creators online and it's my nature to question and flag statistics which don't seem believable. One site reported that epilepsy could be "developed at any time, by any person, of any age, or any stage of life."

*Anyone?* The article pointed out that epilepsy was a disorder, rather than a disease. That made sense to me.

Less than a month later, the second EEG still showed unusual discharges, but I was told the EEG report was returned labelled "normal." My GP suggested no further investigation was required.

Body jerks, I repetitively explained to each new medical professional, or anyone when asked, arrived without warning, and originated from my right lower back. They occurred whenever I stood unsupported and almost immediately when I wasn't grounded by touch or holding on. The strange movements hadn't caused me to lose my balance or fall, though they were disconcerting, and triggered anxious thoughts. A jerk would last no more than a second but would steal my breath away and cause me to emit an *umph* sound, simultaneously. It created a noise like the sound of a speeding ball being caught in a catcher's mitt.

"I'm still having the weird jerks," I repeatedly told my new GP. "What do you think is causing them?" I made appointment after appointment in the hope of understanding and addressing my needs. I tried to be assertive, looking for answers and care. My doctor didn't seem overly concerned.

"Let's wait and see," he said.

My sympathetic nervous system prepared my body for the sudden stress of each jerk, like when someone witnesses a bank robbery in progress and holds tension throughout the incident in anticipation of danger. Typically, my nervous system ought to have made my heartbeat faster to ensure blood was quickly sent to the different body parts that might need it, or cause my adrenal glands to release adrenaline, for a quick getaway. But rather than fleeing in terror, my body jerked.

Usually, our nervous system miraculously controls the body's processes, and we almost never need to think about breathing. At least that's what I'd taught my upper immediate students in science class. Mine appeared to have a few lose connections and to be sending erroneous signals throughout my nervous system.

I continued to jerk about—not something easily explained to friends, supermarket clerks, or total strangers. A similar expression about jerking *off* created vivid images, and laughter, as I attempted to explain my twitchy body. Pretty much everyone who witnessed me jerk in public apologized unnecessarily, thinking that they'd frightened me. It was like when our kids would hide behind their bedroom doors, then jump out and shriek, "BOO!" They were always delighted to startle me.

"Gotcha, Mom." But they hadn't felt the need to apologize. It was all in fun.

The specialist I was first referred to hadn't taken me seriously or listened. He may have been incredibly intelligent, as well as a capable neurologist, but he was equally arrogant and treated me with disdain. He made me feel like I was wasting his precious time. I wasn't impressed. I'd asked my GP for a new referral to someone who could offer a second opinion, and prayed they'd also be skilled at empathy and compassion.

# CHAPTER THREE

### What the Hell Just Happened?

What transpired May 16, 2014, was inconceivable at 7:15 a.m. when I arrived at work.

At fifty, it was twenty-eight years since I'd started my teaching career in Drayton Valley, Alberta. At Courtenay Elementary, in 2013-14, I was in my fifth year of teaching our district's gifted education program and there were only six weeks left in the school year. Students were poised and eagerly discussing their plans for summer vacation. Most school staff members were, too, except the custodial staff for whom summer amounted to the backbreaking labour of cleaning and maintaining the school facility. I had a glimpse into the physical demands of custodial work when, as a university student during the summer of 1983, I worked the 2–10 p.m. shift as one to earn money to complete my degree.

Now, I realized I was running on empty after coordinating and leading a three-day conference for Gifted learners at Mt. Washington Resort. My proverbial batteries needed recharging if I was going to finish the school year strong.

Emotionally drained, I pulled out of the school's staff parking lot. The drive home was a blur. I was appreciative it was a Friday night, and that I'd have the long weekend to unwind. I pressed in our front door's digital key code, unlocked our sanctuary, and sought solace.

Inside, I dropped my phone and keys on the kitchen island's countertop and abandoned my school bag and lunch kit. What I couldn't toss away so easily were my thoughts. They infiltrated my subconscious each waking hour, as well as in my dreams. I often thought about my students on weekends.

I wondered if Sally, one of my current students, would get enough sleep over the weekend while she transitioned back to her mom's house after her parents' recent divorce. With concern, I hoped she took time to play, to lose herself in a fantastical story, feed her insatiable curiosity, and find calm after managing her emotions all day.

Our classroom was an atypical, creative space—some might call unorthodox. It constantly evolved to meet the ever-changing needs of diverse learners. At times it was chaotic, then pulsed back to serene. Challenge, the program I taught, was a pull-out program designated gifted students attended one day each week. Students travelled to Courtenay Elementary and my classroom from across the district and their respective neighbourhood schools for a program specifically targeted to meet the unique, diverse, and complex needs of gifted learners. As their Challenge Teacher, I aimed to establish clear routines, healthy boundaries, and a safe, caring space for my students to learn.

Friday evening, I added crushed ice to my glass, filled it to the brim with Coke Zero, and then slumped into my favourite recliner. I had long since relaxed into the belief that, like the unconditional love from my husband, our strong marriage, and our stable life in the Comox Valley, I was deeply rooted in my chosen career.

Dale would most likely find me seated here when he arrived home from work. I reached out for Dan Brown's latest thriller, bookmarked and inviting, from the side table. I was keen to escape into the questions and curiosity of a murder in Paris's Louvre Museum and its cryptic clues.

With a jolt, my cell phone's ringtone pulled me back to

reality. I jumped up, remembering that I not once, but twice, broke a toe on the corner of our upright grand piano while racing to answer a phone call. Why was it I was always in such a rush? Catastrophizing, as if the world would end if I didn't catch the call.

It was my school's principal, phoning on a Friday night. My intensely busy brain bolted like a rabbit darting to escape a hungry fox.

The week prior I'd asked about spring staffing. Could it happen? Could I lose my treasured position now that I had a continuing contract? There were rumors of deep unexpected layoffs. I worried about a domino effect. Although, I'd been reassured after I heard an implied promise: "We absolutely won't let that happen." I was especially grateful to hear and know this. I believed it.

Now alone, with an anxious heart, I leaned against the island countertop, which divided our open concept kitchen and living room, and listened. My brain was triggered and on full alert. In the past fourteen years, since September 2000, I have held twelve teaching positions in ten different schools and received ten phone calls. Each time I'd get a phone call at the end of May, six weeks before the end of the school year. A call, then pink slip that informed me I'd been laid off.

Ten times, two less than a dozen. Each time I received the proverbial gift – usually a mug with an emblazoned school logo—and was told that I could reapply for yet another teaching position, for the fall term in September.

This year, I believed I was safe. I was secured in a permanent contract, with seniority. I was happily settled in my dream job, confident and anchored. At long last, I'd found my niche. I had a career, a school, a position, and a placement. I was finally enough.

Or was I?

I was, I reassured myself. After twenty-two years of exemplary service, I knew and believed it. Period. No fragments of disbelief. Worthy. I derived profound meaning from the pleasure, support, and esteem my career in gifted education had earned me.

As I held the phone, I reminded myself that I'd earned my position five years earlier. I stopped the anxious thoughts from percolating and took a deep breath. Yet, my mind didn't slow. It raced like a headless chicken. Until again I remembered with gratitude that I was safe. I was tethered and secure. This was just my anxiety getting the best of me. Stop and listen, I told my impulsive self.

Next, through the phone line, I heard words from lips, and knew a mouth was moving. I imagined a facial expression. Circumstances and context were not explained. Year after year, I heard: *It's not personal.* Really? My gut flexed and tightened, and there was a sudden release of energy causing seismic waves that made the ground shake. Nope, it wasn't personal. But embers had been ignited.

After five years, on that Friday night, the phone rang, and again it was *the call*.

"I'm sorry to have to tell you… It's not personal."

News infiltrated, but the trail of words did not. My body understood loss, but my mind did not. A wail pierced the silence. And I realized it was me, as my body folded in on itself and I crumpled to the floor. Frozen, I saw dark edges at the base of the cabinet where my cheek met flooring. I'd heard these words so many times; instinctively I blocked them out. In that instant of realization, something died.

Thoughts invaded: polite, professional leaders listen and respond, someone is still speaking. *You must say goodbye*. Without gathering cohesive thoughts, I heard myself utter, "Goodbye."

*You can hang up now*. I did, and the phone fell to the floor, forgotten.

I was not silent in my weeping. I shrieked with sobs, like a mother who'd given birth to a stillborn. I was speechless with disbelief and loss. My intelligent brain, cognition, and ability to navigate next steps was completely impaired. I was an alcoholic careening along the highway at high speed, oblivious to the impact of my decisions.

Arriving home, my husband saw and reached out for me. With strength, compassion, and love, I was held. Words didn't come. I was empty. Abruptly, I was filled with rage remembering the promise I'd naively trusted. "We absolutely won't let that happen." There would be no tranquility tonight.

What the hell just happened?

JOCELYNBYSTROM

# CHAPTER FOUR

### Biggest Mistake of My Life

*2014*

It's not personal. Are you kidding? Were they #$@!% kidding? These words don't escape my lips after hanging up. Instead, I use my polite, perfectionistic, pleaser's vocabulary, and choose silence. Hatred and emotion are guarded, locked away in the deep recesses of my mind. I don't allow anger, disgust, envy, jealousy, sadness, shame, or guilt to have voices. It isn't safe to do so. Don't be vulnerable, I remind Jocelyn, the wounded child. They'll spot your weaknesses, judge, and find you unworthy.

I'd showed them, all was well.

~

I sat alone, fuming in disbelief through the evening and into the next day. Thinking, I've worked too long, too hard, and proved myself over and over repeatedly. I was so sick of systemic processes deemed humane by a casual acceptance of the status quo. I wanted to screw fear and rant, but I'd learned to protect and defend.

Did they not see my broken-hearted, dispirited body floating? Do they not see me afloat, face down in the wake of their processes? Unlike watercraft that rip past towing water skiers, ski boats leave nothing in their backwash but laughter. I'm barely buoyant and drifting aimlessly in the wake of

Friday's call. Moments last an eternity. Hours seem endless and each is a minefield, for a mind in chaos. Mine, is a mind in peril.

How would I continue to teach with resilience and determination? Perhaps they'd realize they'd made an egregious error and call back, I fantasized. However, my cell phone remained silent. Like me.

Maybe, I'd wake from this nightmare. My mind and subconscious asked endless questions, to which I had no answers.

Were there no witnesses to the long hours I'd worked, or my dedication? Was no one aware I loved my work or that I was honoured to tell others, *teaching gifted education is my calling.* I knew I made a difference and strived tirelessly to meet the needs of each student, cognizant that every student was someone's beloved. I taught them as if they were my own, and nurtured, supported, facilitated, and built relationships with each. My students, their families, and the school community were mine. Now, these had all been ripped away. I hadn't been stabbed in the back; I felt pierced through the heart.

~

I loved school, as a student and as a teacher. I considered myself a lifelong learner. School for me was a haven, a caring, connected community. I loved it. I was grateful for each student, and to work and learn alongside each of my colleagues. As we headed back to school each September, we took great pride in creating inclusive learning communities that embraced diversity, fostered relationships, and empowered every learner.

I believed every child wanted to learn, could learn, and could succeed. With required supports all students could have their needs met at school. Since 1986, I was an educator on a mission and aimed to create classrooms that were welcoming places for my students to wonder, play, create, and build their capacities as leaders, readers, and learners.

~

Saturday, May 17, I was still in a fog of disbelief, teary-eyed and soul-crushed. I was an emotional wreck knowing that I needed to face my students Tuesday morning. Life as I knew it had changed in an instant. One telephone call and my career in gifted education was dead. Something inside of me flatlined.

Death, loss, and grief are universal. When expected or even when unforeseen, we grieve. But this unpredictable loss left me tragically unprepared. Without a roadmap, I couldn't comprehend the how or why. As a child, I managed traumatic incidents through self-control. It was a strategy that once served me well. When insecure or fearful, I controlled my emotions, words, actions, and felt calmer. Safe.

Appearing capable, I believed, made me strong. I continued to use this same strategy into adulthood—to control relationships and unexpected outcomes—and failed.

Without the intrinsic value I equated with my role as a highly specialized leader in my field, I felt vulnerable, naked, and open to attack. I'd been demoted, taken down. My mind reeled in chaos. I was angry and annoyed and wanted to fight.

~

What to do first? I needed to inform parents, I thought. They would want to know. I wanted to relate to each parent, of each of my students from across the district, this bewildering change in leadership. *Why?* I wanted the unexpected news to come through me, so that my students would hear it directly from their parents in my own words, rather than from anyone else. Their parents would help soften, and ease the news, and their grief. I wasn't really thinking clearly. Although, I thought I was.

With the decision to write made, I sat to compose a heart-wrenching letter I cried over as I wrote. I drafted an email hoping to avoid questions Monday morning when astute observant students would read my body language and ask, "What's wrong, Mrs. Bystrom?" I thought a letter of explanation might support parents, as they answered their child's questions. My students were the kinds of kids who would ask the hard questions.

What would I write? I wrote what came to mind and worked diligently to stick to the facts. It was the right thing to do, I believed. I wrote to avoid losing control, falling apart, and crashing in despair Tuesday morning, when after the Victoria Day long weekend, students would be returning to my classroom.

Overwhelmed, I simply couldn't see past my role as Challenge Teacher. I was a specialist, and an integral part of the gifted community. Arrogantly, I believed I was the most qualified individual to meet my students' needs. I was passionate about meeting the unique needs of high-ability learners, and teaching them brought meaning, pleasure, and esteem in this role I'd earned.

I couldn't quite get my head around the loss and swirled in an eddy of grief. All I knew was that I needed to protect myself. A salmon swims upstream to spawn, unaware death awaits. I was suddenly made aware. In shock, I concluded that I was no longer on my chosen career path, and instead, at a dead end.

My heart told me that my students would not want to be blindsided Tuesday morning, as I had been. So, I wrote to protect them, as I would have wanted to be protected. They were vulnerable and at risk, and I didn't want to see them hurt, as I had been.

I wondered if my letter might change anything. I was emboldened by my perception of injustice. I tried to be hopeful.

However, I was extremely naïve.

Teachers hired after January 1, 2001, were laid off the spring of 2014. This included me. I informed parents by email that I would not be returning to my position in September. I explained that based on seniority another teacher would replace me. I asked that parents not come to me with questions, and told them explicitly that if they had questions, the proper protocol was to contact school district personnel or the school board.

This was an error, unbeknownst to me. For ease of communication, I provided contact information. Selfishly, I hadn't wanted to field phone calls, or be contacted by parents with questions, knowing it would cause me further emotional pain. Subconsciously, I wonder if I hoped beyond rationality that the universe would shift and by miraculous intervention the decision to lay me off might be reversed.

After rereading the letter, I'd written, I checked the factual accuracy, corrected typos, and ensured the email addresses I'd included with embedded links were correct. I deemed what I drafted edited and ready. I needed to be certain not to make errors. My intention was to reassure parents, and possibly myself, that all would be well. I hoped it would.

And I pressed, Send.

This action would be the biggest mistake of my life.

~

The parent letter was off into the ether and news of my surprising layoff and reassignment rippled out across the district. In the blink of an eye, my email was also read by administrators. I'd sent them a copy, as was expected. Parents read, families shared, curious children overheard, and my students responded. I received several replies almost immediately, which heartened and lifted my spirits temporarily. Parents responded expressing compassion, surprise, and concern. What I didn't expect, naively, were the immediate repercussions.

I had unknowingly incited action against my employer with my Sunday night email. Action, that I was held responsible for, and to account for after I'd pressed send.

A disciplinary meeting followed May 24, 2014. It caused me inexpressible, irrevocable harm, angst, and trigger as accusatory comments were directed at me. Dormant trauma resurfaced; a letter of direction was written. A letter was placed on my personnel file. I felt labelled and unjustly accused of being highly unprofessional. I managed, barely. The earth's plates moved unknowingly beneath my feet, as they shifted towards one another, ready to collide. An earthquake was imminent.

# CHAPTER FIVE

## If Only

I was raw, suffering in silence. I couldn't tell anyone, not even Dale, that on the inside I was all jagged edges. Prickles and tingling were new sensations. My anxiety magnified and its voice became strong and loud. Still, I didn't want anyone to notice my lost confidence, the powerlessness. Embers of hope grew dim and smouldered, robbing me of joy.

Jarring streaks of bright red and jet black filled my mind, obliterating all beauty and light. Obscured was the blushing innocence of laughter, creativity, and play.

I didn't recognize the urgency of my invisible symptoms. Others didn't either. The seizures weren't happening ... yet.

~

I returned to work in the fall of 2014, after being laid off from my treasured position as Challenge Teacher, with invisible wounds that I worked diligently to conceal while still extremely vulnerable. Internalized loss and grief were effectively burrowing their way into my core.

My return to teaching in a generalist classroom was especially difficult. I'd arrived at a new school and classroom to teach fourth and fifth graders, after being a highly trained, skilled specialist. It felt like a significant step down, and a step that I couldn't really talk about as I joined others who were immersed in this important work as classroom teachers. I was discouraged by individuals that I'd previously considered trusted allies who suggested that I not dwell in my grief, or have a pity party, saying that I wouldn't get what I wanted anyway. To make matters worse, I started in late August amidst stressful, ongoing labor negotiations, and then a full-blown strike.

The school I moved to in 2014-15, espoused Stephen R Covey's ground-breaking leadership, which suggested highly effective leaders were "proactive and took responsibility for their lives, began with the end in mind, and put first things first." Covey elaborated in his school edition version, titled *The Leader in Me*, that effectual facilitators in a school setting followed these same seven habits, slightly modified for the leader in all of us. I buried my unresolved grief and crossed the bridge. I would be an effective leader.

Ironically, walking the picket lines became an unforeseen, helping hand. It provided time and space for me to develop critically important relationships I valued. My colleagues and I literally walked miles and collaboratively carried our collective loads. Day after day during what became a protracted strike, new colleagues welcomed me warmly, which caressed my wounded spirit. By the time classes began in late September, I felt less dispirited and more one of the team.

Month to month, I managed. Teaching in this new role didn't measure up to the role I grieved and festered in me as I tried to embrace the work. I delighted in each new student and derived great pleasure and satisfaction from the privilege to work and learn alongside each of them. But despite putting 110 percent effort into my workday, my heart wasn't fully in the work, as I longed to be back teaching the gifted learners I'd taught in the past.

Initially, I don't think my colleagues or students noticed. I wore masks well. As I taught fourth and fifth graders, I pushed myself with reaching expectations, always expecting exponentially more of myself. *How did other teachers manage?* I wondered as I headed home nearing dinner time, without a planned menu for what to prepare for dinner.

My perfectionistic expectations overwhelmed me in addition to the challenging class dynamics, endless requirements for student assessment, and creation of e-portfolios for each of my students. These in addition to the ever changing and expanding curricular content, which students needed to learn, review and master. How was it possible to keep on top of it all, and still be authentic? I needed to be ready each school day morning with compassion, kindness, and enough energy to teach well-planned and executed lessons. How could I juggle all this and more? I didn't have a clue yet was ashamed to admit my incompetency. I wasn't managing the load but disguised it well. Others even came to me for help. I was a mentor, who supported, encouraged, and trained teachers new to the profession and came alongside others who struggled. It *appeared* all was well.

My best wasn't enough, though. I didn't have more to give. I worked longer hours, and weekends. Dale and I were still best friends, but more like roommates than a true married couple. We tucked in the same bed each night, exhausted and alone. Especially, as I pushed myself towards excellence to regain the labels I needed and constantly strove for: capable, competent, and professional.

I was a hamster on a never-ending wheel who constantly attempted to garner respect, build my resume, and be enough.

I worked to prove my worth constantly. I'd been changed, through repetitive experiences of great loss. Without a roadmap for how to manage stress and grief, I went above, and more often beyond, required expectations in my efforts to build trusted relationships.

I desperately wanted to trust that I'd be warmly welcomed—and able to stay beyond June—however, I no longer trusted the staffing process. The only person I could control was myself. If I worked hard enough, I would prove my value. If I invested an exponential number of hours into nurturing and caring and facilitating student learning, perhaps they'd notice. I imagined, planned, and attempted to create the perfect classroom year after year. But each June, I hadn't succeeded to meet my own expectations.

An empty nester in 2014, I'd supported my students' unmet needs, without attention to my own. I'd parented our children well, I thought. They'd become independent, capable, and kind.

I cared for everyone with compassion and kindness, yet unknowingly became resentful that my efforts didn't yield what I longed for, to believe that others saw me and knew me to be capable and worthy. I craved to belong.

I found it increasingly more difficult to believe that anyone truly knew me or understood my grief. I started to question my own worth as I listened to a critical voice in my head, which replayed damaging words: *You're not smart, you're stupid; you're unprofessional and can't even see, or admit to, your own faults.* I started to believe what wasn't true. The voice was so confident and assured, a bully. I struggled to trust my own instincts and judgement.

How could I prove beyond a shadow of doubt that the words I'd heard, words that shamed, weren't true. I knew they weren't, but couldn't seem to assert myself, or garner support from anyone who I thought believed in me professionally. I threw myself under the bus when I chose not to defend my integrity.

I'd been nominated back during the 2013–2014 school year by over a dozen individuals, including parents of my students, to SENG's Honor Roll, a non-profit network of people who guide gifted, talented, and twice-exceptional individuals to reach their goals intellectually, physically, emotionally, socially, and spiritually. There were letters written nominating me, and I was added to their Honor Roll in 2014. I received an email from SENG (Supporting Emotional Needs of the Gifted), an organization that honoured and labelled me as an educator with "exceptional commitment," and a "special person and champion in the social and emotional development" of others. Which words could I trust? Which were true? These words and labels differed from those which were volleyed across the table at the disciplinary meeting in 2014 and wounded me.

I put heart into the work and arrived home, a broken doll. Work became a blur, and I admitted to a teaching colleague and dear friend that I couldn't pull myself out of the darkness. She presented me with a gift basket of sunshine that overflowed with yellow themed items: balloons, candles, candy, and rays of hope and light, accompanied by a thoughtful card. She saw me and cared. But it wasn't enough. I felt buried, neck deep. The additional burden of my physical deterioration intensified, as did the frequency of jerks.

Over time, a cyclical pattern emerged. I was referred to medical specialists, waited for assessments, and my physical health declined. I'd pressed send, passed go, and repeated the loop around the metaphorical game board. Each year I passed the B&O Railroad and Marvin Gardens, then landed in jail. I didn't have a "get-out-of-jail-free" card. I had to pay the price. It was a time of furrowed brows and unanswered questions. Hurtful words became ticks and burrowed deep.

I prioritized work, my students, their needs, and their families. I prioritized relationships and invested deeply in my new school community. I attempted to do the same at home for Dale, for my mother, and each of my friends. I cared and became a caregiver in each of my valued relationships and prided myself in meeting the needs of others. I prioritized caring despite this adding weight to my already heavily burdened backpack.

~

In the spring of 2016, I was referred to a second neurologist, as well as to the University of British Columbia's Pacific Parkinson's Research Center and movement disorders clinic. Referred to both by my family doctor because, he'd explained, it might be a long wait before either referral was reviewed or appointments were made.

I still hadn't heard back about that 2016 referral to the UBC's Parkinson's clinic by Canada Day 2016. I hoped the neurologist specializing in what ailed me would give the office clerk the nod soon.

Perhaps my file was embedded in a deep stack of dormant medical records, electronically tucked away in a forgotten folder labelled, Not Yet. Did someone need to give someone in the know the nod and signal another to pick up my file?

Did another Parkinson's patient need to die to create an opening in my specialist's caseload? Would my mind and body expire because of a serious underlying undiagnosed illness, while I waited? I asked myself in the mirror, *Do I have Parkinson's?*

My psyche needed a diagnostic label, even if a label meant a diagnosis of Parkinson's, a cancerous brain tumor, or MS (multiple sclerosis). Fearing that I had a life-shortening disease made matters worse.

I heard the telltale clunk of the letter box lid July 2, 2016. I reached in and dimples erupted with my smile as I read the easily identifiable postmark. I opened the letter from UBC's Parkinson's clinic with great anticipation, my pupils scanning for an appointment date. "July 28" caught my eye.

*That wasn't so long to wait,* I'd thought. *Just over three weeks.*

I could hold on knowing I'd be seeing a specialist in just twenty-six days. Then my grey-matter signalled an autocorrect. I smiled right up until I reread the appointment date more closely: July 27, 2017.

There'd be another year of waiting.

I'd noted the detail I searched for, but not the year. July 28, *2017,* was bolded further down the page. I'd need to wait another twelve months. *It couldn't be, could it?* It must be a mistake.

I called to confirm. It wasn't an error.

We rang in the new year, January 1, 2017, and the official countdown to my appointment began. Only 208 days to go. My body needed to be weaned off antiepileptic medications, and I learned it would be an almost three-month long process. My body doesn't adapt well to adjustments or changes to medication, so my family doctor reduced the dosages very slowly over a longer period to eliminate any residual medication in the hope of minimizing undesirable side effects.

I could star in my own Hollywood production of *Freaky Friday*. I was to present my fabulously freaky body which jerked every few seconds as I stood unsupported off meds at my July 27 appointment. The jerks surprised specialists. Unusual and rare were both words used to describe my odd symptoms at that appointment. Myoclonic jerks weren't rare, but the way mine presented was unique. They asked my permission to record video for medical research purposes. Chuckling, my neurologist at the UBC Parkinson's clinic, a specialist in neuromuscular disorders, commented with a grin, "You'll be a star, but sadly, the movie won't be syndicated, streamed on Netflix, or pay royalties."

Dale and I were impressed by the thoroughness of the investigations at that initial appointment. First, I'd been assessed by a neurologist, training alongside the movement-disorder neurologist, and then again by Dr. Silke Creswell, the neuro-muscular neurologist specialist I'd waited a year to see. She'd completed her own thorough exam. Finally, the two highly intelligent, skilled neurologists collaborated as mentee and mentor. Dale and I listened intently. Their relationship was an exceptional example of everything I'd learned about mentor-protégée relationships in the workplace. There was evidence of collaboration and trust. It was apparent to both Dale and I that both doctors experienced mutual benefits and satisfaction from their relationship, conversations, and collaboration.

Ultimately, I thought, I would be the benefactor of their shared expertise. I was mesmerized by Dr. Creswell's intelligence and aptitude as a diagnostician. It was easy to feel reassured and trust my health and wellness were safely in the hands of experts.

Afterwards, I'd read Dr. Creswell's online bio, and was not surprised to learn she was both an internationally recognized speaker for her work on Parkinson's research, as well as the founding director of the BC Brain Wellness Foundation. During that first appointment with Dr. Creswell, my gut told me I could trust her care, insights, and well-articulated expertise. But, I'd wondered, *Do I have Parkinson's disease?*

As Dale and I exited the elevator and walked hand in hand back to our parked vehicle I couldn't help but be curious about why I'd been specifically referred to the Pacific Parkinson's Research Center?

Had my GP, or the locum, suspected something and not told me?

I was extremely grateful for my appointment with Dr. Creswell, after experiencing two previous neurologists who'd insinuated there was no physical evidence underlying the symptoms I described and implied that my physical symptoms were all in my head. *I am not a liar.*

Both Dale and I commented as we unlocked our parked car that we'd each experienced a spark of hope after I'd received this measure of clarity, a likely diagnosis, and a new forward-thinking treatment plan.

Dr. Creswell had said, "Based on our observations and assessments today, it's most likely that you have propriospinal myoclonus (PSM), a rare neurological disorder with repetitive, usually brief jerks of the trunk, hips, and knees in a fixed pattern."

It hadn't been all in my head.

~

Jerks diagnosed and labelled "myoclonic jerks" continued after Dr. Creswell prescribed a new medication called clonazepam. Dr. Creswell understood that I needed to titrate up slowly on any new medication after I'd told her of my past challenges with new medications. She recommended that I take my time and titrate up on the new medication similarly to how I came off the valproic acid for my initial appointment with her.

Between the heat of summer and Christmas the frequency of symptoms varied. I kept in touch with Dr. Creswell by phone, and she'd prescribed a substitute when clonazepam produced excessive drowsiness and cognition challenges. It was difficult to work during these medication trials, however I had. Next, she prescribed Keppra in September 2017. It similarly caused disconcerting side effects, including mood changes and irritability. Side effects continued to outweigh the benefits of new and varied medications, and in October Dr. Creswell had me return to valproic acid, the antiepileptic I was on successfully prior to investigations at the Parkinson's Research Center. I was grateful for her willingness to be called upon during these experimental trials of new medications, and her trust and compassion of my intuition and intelligence, when I announced, "I need to stop taking clonazepam."

She listened.

Thankfully the return to the valproic acid helped without the aggressive side effects I'd experienced on the other meds. I also continued taking Wellbutrin for generalized anxiety. Who wouldn't be anxious I thought, after all these varied drug trials?

By January 1, 2018, I could no longer stand unsupported without jerks occurring every few seconds. Dr. Creswell had planted the seed that I consider either a rolling walker or a cane back in July.

Wait, what? I'd just turned fifty. I don't need mobility aides, I'd stubbornly thought. But without support for stability, and too proud to use a cane or walker, I endured frequent, intense jerks that aggravated my already sore body between July and December. It became a vicious cycle of jerks and chronic pain. Just before I attended first the local Remembrance Day Parade, and then my previous school's Christmas concert, I purchased myself a cane. It was tougher than swallowing a pill. Showing up using a cane made my invisible disability all too visible.

Continued evidence on successive EEGs of epileptiform spikes and discharges ensured I was kept under scrutiny and prompted additional medications. With each new drug there were two parts of the equation to balance—symptoms with side effects. What dosage was necessary to reduce symptoms, which were constantly increasing in frequency, intensity, and duration; and minimize brutal side effects. It was a constant struggle to find an equilibrium. My body didn't adjust easily, and dark circles appeared beneath puffy eyelids.

Eleven months later, in November 2018, I returned to UBC for a follow-up with Dr. Creswell, my neuromuscular neurologist.

To reach appointments at the UBC clinic required we leave the Comox Valley, drive one and a half hours to Nanaimo, and wait in line for the next available departure on BC Ferries. Then there would be a ninety-minute crossing of the Strait of Georgia before the ferry docked in Horseshoe Bay. It would take another sixty-minute commute after disembarking the ferry before we'd reach the UBC campus and appointment. That was if there were no accidents or traffic jams.

We typically headed over the night before the appointment, leaving after Dale and I finished work, to ensure we reached the mainland from Vancouver Island with certainty. Storms blow up unexpectedly, the ferry can be cancelled without notice. When you've waited months, or even years, for an appointment you make darn sure you don't miss it due to inclement weather. An overnight stay can also be required for the return trip home dependent on the timing of my appointments and availability of return departures on BC Ferries. Travelling to appointments with specialists in the lower mainland meant long, exhausting days for both my medical escort—usually Dale—and me.

Dale repeatedly took time off work to attend my appointments and travel to Vancouver from Comox. We were both anxious for clarity and understanding. Although I could still drive myself in 2018, and travel alone, I often asked Dale to accompany me. I needed his emotional support. He grounded me and brought calm to an otherwise anxiety-producing appointment and journey.

I was re-evaluated November 2, 2018, at UBC's Parkinson's Research Center. Again, first by another neurologist and new protégée working alongside Dr. Creswell.

In collaboration, they changed my diagnosis. At the end of my second appointment at UBC, I was diagnosed with orthostatic myoclonus, and referred to yet another neurologist. My curious brain was intrigued while my anxious brain worried. The new specialist suggested electromyography tests and nerve conduction studies as well as a modified treatment plan. My intelligent brain, Googled.

~

Teachers, like medical practitioners, are one of several helping professions prone to burnout. Having taught in at least ten different schools, I can say with confidence, teachers care deeply about their work. There may be the odd exception, but as a rule my colleagues through my years demonstrated empathy and kindness beyond measure. I, too, cared deeply about my students and their learning.

Educators, like health care professionals, are at risk of compassion fatigue. Self-care ought to be a key part of the mental health conversation in our workplaces, but this wasn't my experience between 1986–2018. Educators provide emotional labor; we know ours is a helping profession. The demands of the role itself are not for the faint of heart, or salary driven individuals. No one I knew, voluntarily, spoke of their inability to meet the demands of the ever- increasing workload and challenging expectations, especially at work. Perhaps in hushed tones, the courageous might confide that they're struggling, but I hadn't heard any such whispers. Had anyone else struggled in silence as I did?

When my colleagues and I gathered for a rare after-work social, there may have been occasional grumbles about being over-tired, and not enough hours in the day. Or the odd "That really made me mad" story. But more often we'd lift each other up with encouragement. It takes self-discipline and practice to turn off your teacher brain. I'm guessing many, like me, went home too tired to prioritize their needs… and their teacher brain continued to crank out unwanted thoughts.

I jokingly told myself, and others, that I was a recovering perfectionist, as I attempted to ensure my lengthy to-do list got accomplished. No matter how many hours I put into checking off items, there was always more to do. I couldn't keep ahead of the list. Had my list differed from that of others providing emotional labour? I didn't think so. Employees in the public sector and helping professions seem to be constantly expected to do more with less. Each time I was praised for accomplishing more (with less), it seemed the expectation increased once again. If only I worked harder and longer, perhaps I'd complete more. What I had to offer, with the amount of energy I could muster, never seemed enough. I couldn't seem to meet the students' needs for connection, safety, and belonging, in addition to mastery of grade level expectations. I couldn't keep abreast of the latest technology, support the school community, coach after-school clubs, attend needed professional development to confidently manage expectations AND balance it all with living. The written and unwritten expectations—whether imposed by others, the employer, or myself—were tough to manage. Add in the hopes of students' families, the school district, the government (a.k.a. your employer), keep abreast of current trends and best practices in teaching, and manage through an unexpected global pandemic. It's too much, and I was not enough.

What could I let go of? What if I got caught prioritizing what others believed was optional and/or unnecessary? Or inversely what if I hadn't prioritized what was an expected given? What if my students didn't meet grade level expectations through no fault of their own or mine? What if test results on the FSA or standardized testing made me look bad as a teacher? I did my best. What if that wasn't enough. What if parents, the employer, and my colleagues who'd admired me, found out that I was in fact unprofessional and an imposter. I wasn't unprofessional or an imposter, however I'd started believing I might be, and shame made me see my abilities in a negative light that ate away at my confidence. Despite frequent reassurances that I was competent and highly professional, none of it mattered because I didn't believe it.

Expectations I layered on my own shoulders were multiplied by students, their parents, administrators, curricular expectations, new trends and technology, changing assessment practices, as well as by societal change and the employer. Was I surprised that my body was keeping score? Yes.

I didn't see any correlation.

Who had time to do the math? Does anyone keep tabs on an emotional labourer's emotional regulation? I didn't have time for reflection. I was too busy surviving my load as I trudged uphill.

~

My classroom each year, was often populated by an ever-increasing cast of children, arriving with unmet needs and telling behaviors. Children, who arrived for an 8:30 a.m. start-up whose behaviour attempted to speak of perhaps an underlying lack of security, stability, consistency, emotional support, love, structure, and /or positive role models. It was heart-wrenching at times to witness my student's vulnerability and neediness.

I successfully worked four days a week, with a doctor's mandated rest day, Wednesdays. This mid-week break intended for my body to recuperate from the myoclonic jerks was often used to chip away at my to-dos. I learned about mindfulness, even taught mindfulness to students. However, I hadn't known how to create calm for myself. For three years I worked four days a week, with a supposed day of rest. I rested rarely.

Again, in 2018, my neurologist recommended a change just after fall start-up. I'd needed her permission, and a decision was made on my behalf when I was no longer capable of making it for myself. I needed to take small but necessary steps to prioritize care for myself. She recommended a full, rather than increased partial, leave. With an extremely heavy heart, I said goodbye to students and colleagues I was attached to. It had become a vicious cycle.

After the significant loss of my career in gifted education in 2014, I was traumatized.

A second, part-time medical leave, blindsided me. I hadn't seen it coming. It was both a physical and emotional necessity. It would be a leave that retriggered childhood strategies, without appropriate tools for coping with additional losses. I was pulled out of my classroom mid-year after a neurologist explained the necessity. I managed.

For my third leave of absence, also full-time, I was placed on long-term-disability from November 2018 to June 2019. This time I saw it coming. I was struggling physically, relationally, and emotionally.

At the end of June 2019, and after a full year dedicated to health and wellness, and prioritizing self-care, I finally felt ready to return to work for the first time in years. I'd retrained as a teacher-librarian and felt physically strong again. There'd been fewer residual myoclonic jerks after another medication change to Brivlera. I felt good. I was strong.

~

Figuratively, I geared up in my paddling gear, jumped in my kayak, and scouted the current downstream, as years ago I was a strong white-water paddler and enthusiast. I knew these muddied waters on the river ahead, filled with rocks, eddies, and turbulence. I knew I'd meet conscientious, well-outfitted, adventurous paddlers along the way who'd coursed downstream on similar journeys ill-equipped. I trusted there would be skilled mentors and instructors to teach and aide me in the hopes that I'd be able to courageously proclaim my beliefs, values, and priorities. I'd chosen to acknowledge the One to whom I belonged, the Good Shepherd, and my rock years ago. He would be my guide, and in control. Not I.

With the sun at my back, Dale at my side, we paddled down river reminiscent of the expeditions of our youth. Prayerfully protected, we threw our heads back, and laughter slipped out effortlessly. I anticipated the joy of the flow ahead.

I wanted to be brave and to glow in this sweet spot, I'd believed truth.

Instead, I'd imagined with certainty the rapids, the barrel and drop over the falls. If only someone had noticed. Instead, I braced for the decent.

JOCELYN BYSTROM

# CHAPTER SIX

## Fractured Bedrock

Slowly, over a long period, a geological fault had formed since shortly before my second birthday. At a time when my mother fearfully left my father, after he'd come home drunk again and accidentally lit the marital bed on fire.

A fault, along which there would be simultaneous, and incremental geological forces: an alcoholic father who abandoned parental responsibility, a traumatized single mother, unmet emotional needs, and constant fear. There would be displacement of plates, which included frequently moving to new communities, arriving in each with a desire for a forever friend, and an introduction to new caregivers while Mom worked twelve-hour shifts. Each year, there was fracturing of bedrock: leaving a neighborhood where I felt safe, leaving a bedroom I loved, and another new best friend. Rocks disintegrated under strain, with constant pressure changes throughout adolescence, and as a young adult.

Newlyweds in 1983, Dale and I left the community where we'd attended high school, met, and married, and where both our parents lived. We left Evansburg, Alberta to pursue our dreams and adventure. We moved to Edmonton, where I completed a teaching degree in 1986, at the University of Alberta.

Afterwards, Dale and I returned to Evansburg, where I taught for five years, and he rejoined the family business;

JALA Ridge Plumbing and Heating. In 1991, Dale and I moved to British Columbia, as adventurous hearts and even bigger dreams led us to the west coast of Vancouver Island. Dale chose to leave the family business after I got a teaching position in the small coastal village of Tahsis. It was an important choice we made together, and it felt right. It was not a simple choice, and we'd later learn there would be repercussions.

There was more seeking, starting over, and sending down tender roots. Shortly after we moved to the remote community of Tahsis, Dale's dad, who'd been terminally ill, died just six months after we left Evansburg in 1992. His parents had chosen not to tell us. We later learned they'd hoped Dale would take over the family business.

There was guilt and shame after leaving. We hadn't been told of Dale's dad's critical health, and I wondered why they felt it needed to be a secret. They'd let us go, move away, and make an uninformed decision. A gift, I thought earlier but was it? Regret left us raw and in pain, which wasn't easy to talk about. I internalized the pain and grief. I believed both Dale and I did. It wasn't talked about.

Dale's father had longed to be a grandpa during our eleven-year marriage and didn't hold back making this known. We married in 1983 when Dale was twenty-one and I was just nineteen. We'd both known what we wanted. Dale had asked me to be his wife weeks after we'd started dating. My answer had been an easy one. "Of course," I said.

After the wedding had come and gone. Arne, Dale's dad, lovingly began saying, "You've practiced enough." The implication was clear. He, too, knew what he wanted.

As I observed Dale's family life with two parents, and his many relatives with strong, stable marriages, I'd known what *I* wanted. I wanted to ensure we had a strong, stable marriage before we had children. I feared becoming a single mother, as mine had, after witnessing how hard her struggle had been. Despite our strong marriage, I didn't want to have children until we both agreed the right time had arrived. It was important to not find myself with teenaged children, and a husband who might say, you're the one who wanted kids, you deal with it. Dale hadn't ever uttered such a comment, but I imagined the possibility and catastrophized. Dale had never given me any reason to think he would ever act this way. It seemed an innate fear.

We weren't ready for kids, so we waited. Our just right timing, however, filled us with regret after his dad's death, at having not fulfilled Arne's wishes to be a granddad.

When in 1993, we did at last choose to prepare for children and I went off the pill, it wasn't long till I was expecting. I literally jumped up in the air and clicked my heels with excitement after taking the pregnancy test. Dale and I believed like most first-time parents we'd given birth to the most amazing, brilliant, beautiful child ever in 1994, and then two. A son, and then a daughter two years later.

"Congratulations, you have a daughter," the nurse told me in August 1996 after what was an extremely intense, frightening labor and delivery. It had differed completely from the first, a C-section. We were delighted, but she cried twenty-four seven. Everywhere we went, people stared and asked, "Have you thought about using a soother?" Little did they know I'd purchased eight different brands. None helped. They didn't know the big picture, nor did we. I didn't have the energy to explain. Even Dale, while we'd been on a ten-hour road trip to visit dear friends and show them our beautiful new baby girl, Kristen, had asked for divine intervention: "Please God, let the screaming stop."

Illegally, I'd taken Kristen out of her car seat and held her to my breast, nursing for the duration of the road trip. Nothing else worked. I was beyond exhausted, felt judged by passersby, and worried constantly as I imagined us in an auto-accident, and the worst-case scenario occurring. In horror, I realized the truth we would have to live with. Crying and self-judgement continued, and our baby girl cried too. Even when a doctor gave us a prescribed medication to help her wee body get some rest, and said, "Don't be afraid if she sleeps for several hours," she'd only slept for ten minutes. Those years as a new mom were a blur of cuddling, playing, singing love songs to our two sweeties, and falling asleep on the couch while both were within reach. I knew I couldn't keep my eyes open another second and prayed, "Please Lord, take care of them, I cannot." Alarmed, I had awakened with a telltale head jerk and judged myself harshly. Though grateful for a few minutes of rest, I appreciated social services would never know, and the statute of limitations for child neglect has long passed. Our children, now in their mid-twenties, survived into adulthood, and still tell me I'm loved. They told me recently that I'm a great mom. Some days I believe it's true.

There had been parenting without extended family nearby until my mom retired to the Comox Valley in 1998. As well as returning to work after staying at home with our young children at a time when teaching positions were extremely difficult to earn, there were constant layoffs from temporary postings, and an overarching inability to re-establish professional roots and security, after having had a continuing contract and security in Alberta, and British Columbia prior to having our children. It was tough to go back to work when I wanted to after taking time off to parent our young children.

Our daughter blessed us beyond measure. Eventually, we found out why she cried endlessly. Our general practitioner, who I deeply respected, and who had delivered Kristen, suggested we take her to a chiropractor. What? I thought. Take my newborn to a bone cruncher? I did not understand chiropractic work and had only heard talk of bones being adjusted and cracking and joints popping. I imagined it was excruciatingly painful. My doctor went on to explain recent research where babies who endured traumatic births were being successfully treated by chiropractors, and it might be worth our consideration. I was desperate, so didn't consider long. I telephoned and made an appointment ASAP with the chiropractor she'd recommended. Dale, Keith, our dog Buffy, and I were all eager to enjoy a quiet, happily content newborn. There must be an underlying need. We hoped the chiropractor could identify what it was. Perhaps finally, she would have relief for whatever it was she so desperately tried to communicate.

When the date of the chiropractic appointment arrived, Keith, then two and a half, and I, put our crying bundle of pink sweetness into her car seat, and headed out full of hope. Keith, always curious, was fascinated despite his crying sister, by the aquarium in the doctor's office. While we waited, he asked questions and commented on many unique characteristics of each fish. "Look Mom, diagonal stripes." Heading into the treatment room directed by the receptionist, Kristen settled momentarily. She was swaddled and immobilized in my arms as we waited for the chiropractor to arrive.

When he arrived, he asked about Kristen's birth and delivery. He then explained that before he initially assessed her, he would explain how the rest of this appointment would go. He wouldn't proceed with treatment unless he could identify something specific that required care, reassuring me that if he found nothing, he would not treat or do anything experimentally. If after today's examination I decided I wanted to proceed, it would be normal and expected to want to leave, think it over, and discuss it with my partner. "Husband," I interjected. I've always been proud to be Dale's wife. The chiropractor offered I could phone his receptionist if we wanted to proceed with treatment and make a follow-up appointment.

I told him I was ready and wanted her to have an initial assessment today, immediately. I didn't need more time to think or to discuss it further with anyone. Go ahead with the initial assessment I repeated. "Are you sure?" he asked.

"Absolutely!" As I passed our beloved newborn to him, she cried. Her legs momentarily dangled after I unwrapped her from the receiving blanket and passed her fragile body to him. Ever so gently, he placed her tiny body on the treatment table, holding her securely and cradling her neck. I was calm and curious. He used his fingers to cradle her fragile body and his thumbs to caress her back ever so lightly, like a gentle tickle or soft whisper. It seemed he hardly touched her at all. His assessment was over quickly, and he carefully lifted and returned Kristen to me. As I held her, she cried, as usual. To hear the doctor more easily, I tucked her into her car seat and monitored both Keith and Kristen, hands free, prepared as possible to listen.

The chiropractor noted and identified a couple of places on Kristen's spine that could benefit from change. Change meant a chiropractic adjustment. Not *might* help but *could*. He felt confident there had been injury, which was likely causing pain whenever she moved and making her cry. It made sense to this exhausted mom. When Kristen was at my breast or swaddled, she was immobilized, and without pain. She didn't need to cry. Alternately, any time we rocked, or jiggled, or attempted to soothe her, she cried out as if to say, "Stop moving me!" . . . except that all we heard was endless crying. Injuries to her neck and back were most likely sustained during her delivery when the umbilical cord had been wrapped around her neck—a crisis which needed for her to be delivered with extreme haste.

Again, the chiropractor recommended taking time to think over the treatment decision. He didn't realize I'd already done so on the spot. To proceed or not to proceed. A question easily answered.

What was there to think about? My daughter was in agonizing pain and had been for months. Every time her precious, fragile body moved, it was excruciatingly painful. "Please treat her immediately. Today."

"Are you sure?"

Why does he keep asking? I wondered. If he could take her pain away, why wait. "Please treat her immediately," I almost begged.

"Alright then, this won't take long." This, as I pressed Kristen back into his arms and my heart leapt ignited by a spark of hope. An answer to my prayers seemed possible. *Please, Dear Lord...* I prayed while he worked.

He placed Kristen carefully back down on the table as I watched. Mesmerized by his fingers and thumbs, I watched as he manipulated my precious daughter's tiny body. I'd given him permission and was completely exhausted. I hadn't been thinking clearly enough to be fearful. What he did looked like nothing more than thumbs gently massaging. There was no crunch, no sound, and it had been unlike anything I imagined. I was grateful and relieved. It was over in seconds, and he passed her back.

"That's all for today. Make another appointment for early next week. Call and let me know how she's doing. And if you have questions, just call." Keith, understanding that the appointment was over, headed out of the small room a few steps ahead of me, in anticipation of needing quiet. He and I both knew what to expect as I lovingly tucked Kristen into her car seat.

Except it didn't happen. Keith looked up at me, clearly surprised, his head tilted before raising his eyebrows. I reached for his hand, then reached back for the handle of Kristen's car seat as we headed to the receptionist's desk. As we left, I peered down, and a smile instinctively spread across my face. Our sweet baby girl was silent, and her eyelids fluttering.

I was baffled, elated, and overwhelmed with gratitude simultaneously. My joy increased as I realized the miraculous nature of what had just occurred. As I made the follow-up appointment, I noticed Keith pointing into the car seat. Kristen had fallen asleep. "Look Mom, she's tired." So was I—exhausted yet happy.

"Let's go to the bakery and celebrate." Keith chose a giant chocolate chip cookie, and I ordered him a small milk, and then ordered myself a cup of tea. Maybe, just maybe, Kristen would nap long enough for me to enjoy it.

I had nothing to worry about; my infant daughter slept soundly for six hours; pain free at last. She hadn't wakened for the car trip home, going into the house, or when I moved her to her crib. I kept checking every few minutes to make sure she was still breathing. She was. But still I had to check. I could hardly wrap my exhausted brain around what had transpired. Who knew tiny babies experienced trauma during delivery? We bonded over shared trauma, hers and mine.

Thank goodness she could communicate her need for help. Thank God she persisted and advocated for her needs. And that she wasn't willing to take no for an answer. She had cried for good reason. Thank goodness, we listened. Why couldn't we have learned sooner. Thank goodness, my doctor, despite nearing retirement, was humble and receptive, with a growth mindset to new research and changing medical strategies to promote wellness. Her willingness to suggest a novel intervention literally saved me and saved us.

We'd been mightily blessed. Our kids seemed typical, though I hadn't grown up around many children. Most of my experiences with children were lived second-hand through the students I taught at school. I had little to no understanding of what to expect from my own. Unlike Dale, who grew up surrounded by cousins, many aunts and uncles, and a significant extended family, I had an extended family of three: Aunty Peggy, Uncle Harry, and Grandpa, Mom's dad. And we didn't see them frequently, as they didn't live nearby. There were others I wasn't aware of, but for reasons unknown or not shared by Mom, they didn't seem connected through my prized childhood kaleidoscope.

Unlike my childhood, our children Keith and Kristen were surrounded with extended family as they grew up. Dale's family, were now mine. Ours.

*What's his was mine, right?* I'd won the jackpot, after saying, "I do."

"Mommy, if God created the earth in seven days, why did

the dinosaurs live long before animals existed in the creation story?" asked Keith, at three. I learned quickly to defer to mentors, redirect to research, seek expertise, and attempt to find age-appropriate answers. Responses which would satisfy his insatiable demand for knowledge and understanding. By four, we thought it funny when he lay on the top bunk and read novels. We hadn't realized he was indeed reading. At bedtime Keith memorized stories, and knew them well enough that one day, while at the public library for Children's Story Hour, he rudely interrupted the librarian. While she read aloud, he'd felt it important to inform her, "You've made a reading error." Arne, not Tact, is Keith's middle name. My cheeks were instantaneously a deep red, though the librarian didn't skip a beat. She made a brief comment I don't remember, and carried on, undeterred. The littles gathered around hadn't a clue. I reminded myself to have a serious chat with our son about tact and diplomacy, interrupting others, and manners. I believed his behaviour reflected on me. She'd judged me for it, and others would too. My mother taught me well. I needed to keep up appearances.

With legs that dangled from the shopping cart, Keith, at five, sat mesmerized, unaware of gawking strangers in the grocery aisles. As I strolled up and down, shopping list in hand, Keith was absorbed in Harry, Hagrid, and Dumbledore's antics and spells. He was oblivious to Frosted Flakes, Oreos, or the harsh comment someone felt it necessary to share directed at me for "letting my young son read such a book." This, as we shopped for apples and bananas. Somehow, he would always pull himself out of the trance as we reached the bakery. He remembered kids received a free cookie, and that he wanted one. Afterwards, we reversed direction and went back to check the produce off the grocery list.

Our children loved books. Cuddling with our precious two reading their chosen favourites filled me with joy. We read together each night. It was our bedtime routine, not unlike many parents with children ages five and three. Occasionally, as I tucked Keith in, we would read a novel side by side. I would read aloud, unknowing he had already read ahead. I learned only as I read, and his smirk and sparkling eyes provided clues. He already knew what was about to happen. Later that evening, with my bedside reading light poised, I attempted to read late into the night, hoping to catch up and get ahead. I turned off the light, thinking I had. Had I? I hadn't.

I tried to remember if my mom had cuddled with us at bedtime. Had she read to us? I couldn't remember. I didn't ask when I might have. Now I cannot. In 2021, her words and stories have been silenced by dementia. I'll never know. Of one thing I was certain, I valued reading and cuddling. Had she been too tired or working late? I have so very many questions, like our young son.

Keith left me in the dust, reading beyond what I had time to keep up with. It was then I realized my role had shifted. I became his facilitator of reading and learning. He was in the driver's seat. Lesson #1–I was not in control; yet I thought I was and wanted to be. I taught our children to choose books, novels, and non-fiction that felt just right for their needs. I hoped they would find the "just right books" that, as voracious readers, wouldn't get them in over their heads.

Just because a child can read doesn't mean you want your five-year-old accidentally reading content with explicit violence or sex. Nope, save that for when they're six. I was ever on the hunt for the elusive engaging story, or non-fiction text, with an intriguing plot, meaty enough to pique Keith's interests. Who is this kid, with the endless questions? Was Dale like this when he was a kid? I wondered. And then I realized I missed Keith's reliance on me. He became independent too soon. I missed that sweet little boy who reached up for me, smiling and longing to be cuddled, nurtured, and supported. It's what I needed and craved still.

Each unmet need took a toll and caused further erosion of my armature.

By the time Keith was thirteen in 2007, I had worked my way through several full-time, temporary contracts. Parents are their children's first and fiercest teacher and advocate. I loved books and regarded them as treasures with answers. My brain was filled with so very many questions, and certainly not enough answers. I needed books. Nowhere, it seemed, to this mother of two, was there the parenting manual I needed. Where was the copy of Heidi Murkoff's *What to Expect When Your Children Are Eleven and Thirteen*? You know Murkoff's long overdue sequel to *What to Expect When You're Expecting*, which I lapped up with ravenous thirst throughout my first pregnancy. When I couldn't find answers, I lost sleep.

With a brain on fire, gears grinding, and constant shifting, I worried when I ought to have been recharging my batteries. Awake, I puzzled over unanswered questions. If only I'd been able to ask Siri, or Google. Keith had a mind of his own, which was a good thing. I knew that. However, I hopelessly longed to understand the inner workings of his mind. I desperately wanted to love him fully and felt incompetent. It was far too soon to cut the apron strings, so I kept the scissors tucked safely away in my sewing kit.

Meanwhile, I went back to school, earned a master's degree in educational leadership and counselling, with a research focus on gifted education. When I completed my degree in 2009, I was delighted to leave both the generalist classroom and temporary contracts behind, which had me teach every grade—kindergarten through ninth—and move into my new role as Challenge Teacher. The stars had aligned, and I finally earned a full-time, continuing contract.

Teaching gifted learners, like our own children, was deeply satisfying. I connected to this community, and it seemed I innately belonged. Students roared with excitement like a crowd cheering on their favourite driver at the Indy 500. Every hand was raised with curiosity, intention, and passion. Each student dared to take learning risks, corners at speed, and make mistakes as they rubbed fenders with other drivers on the track. This, as they experienced the thrill of autonomous learning, a track where divergent, convergent, and critical thinking were expected, and students pushed themselves to their outer limits. Because it was the expected norm and part of the thrill as you put on your helmet, buckled up before the flashing reds disappeared, and green signaled, Go.

This work, which I enjoyed between 2009–2014 gave me the same high I imagined my husband would get if offered the chance to drive a single seat, open-cockpit, open-wheeled race car with substantial front and rear wings and its high-performance engine at his back. He'd jump at the chance to drive in a Formula One Grand Prix event. I was in the fast lane in 2014, in gear, revved up, and ready to go. Then out of the blue, I was D.N.F.—Disqualified, and Did Not Finish, as they say in Formula One.

Our daughter also blessed us beyond measure as she grew and developed. Her smile lit up any room. It filled me. I hadn't realized two children as different as night and day could be brother and sister, and from the same gene pool. Kristen loved drama, musicals, and enjoyed singing and playing various instruments. Our home in Comox, where I was now deeply rooted after living since 1994, was filled with love, laughter, and music while our kids grew up. I had incredible gratitude for the music they shared, as well as for the laughter they brought into our home.

My mom hadn't laughed. Life was serious, and she took it seriously. When I joined Dale's family, I struggled to understand the humor in the jokes they constantly shared. Humor, it seemed, was like a foreign language. After someone would tell a joke, I'd lean into Dale's side and whisper, "Can you explain that to me?" He would, after I prodded, or later when we got home. Sometimes, he would chuckle, and say, "You don't really want to know." He was right. Sometimes they told raunchy jokes, which made me super uncomfortable. Back to my family. Any dialogue about sexuality, intimacy, or the human body seemed taboo. We never spoke of it. It didn't take long to adapt, and love Dale's big boisterous family that shared openly. I soon realized what I had missed out on.

Kristen in 2009, then in her teens, would go bananas over pi, though not banana cream, blackberry, or peach. She was a mathematician at heart and set her sights early on becoming an actuary. At twelve, she told me her life goals, and of her desire to be a mother, and that she wanted children. Undeterred by obstacles, Kristen studied and worked diligently through high school to achieve her goals. It constantly surprised me how wise and mature our kids had become so quickly. Much to my surprise and dismay, I would later learn Kristen was not as resilient as she appeared, much like her mama, and her grandma.

JOCELYN BYSTROM

# PART TWO

## SEASON OF REFLECTION

JOCELYN BYSTROM

# CHAPTER SEVEN

### Mom's Story, A Fractured Fairy Tale

"Mom, don't forget to use your words," I almost beg her in 2021. Occasionally, her brain surprises and delights. Just when I think she's about to express something, she cannot. This isn't new. Now the inhibition is because of physical changes in her brain, and frontal temporal dementia. Already acclimated from childhood, I still long for Mom to be in front of me with a voice and words of affection.

"I need…." she utters.

I'd forgotten Mom's last few precious phrases. I am overwhelmed with emotion, always hanging on her words, and wishing she would complete her sentences. Any expression which might help me know *what* she needs, or wants, is a rare occurrence. I long to hear "I love you" before it is too late. These words, the ones I need to hear, are no longer in her vocabulary. Perhaps, it *is* too late. It's been too late for a lifetime. Now, she doesn't remember my name, or that I'm her daughter. She thanks me often for being good to her, which is enough. It's what she can give.

A beauty, but unlike Marilyn Monroe. My mother, Sydney, is not sexy-beautiful, but a classic beauty. When I was a child, she was elegant, poised and held herself like Grace Kelly or Audrey Hepburn with movie star's good looks. That was then. More recently, her resilient beauty cheats time without plastic surgery. In 2014, Mom's skin still glowed and very few wrinkles disguised her near eighty years. Her mind was still sharp, an expected Hall family trademark, although she'd married into these expected norms. Hers would not be the journey she expected through aging. Mom's face, at eighty-three, remains classic, recently framed with delicate folds like a lovely silk scarf. Maps and stories of wisdom and the joys of grandchildren are now etched deeper by weight loss.

"I'm just not hungry anymore. I'm sorry." She believes she's offended me when she doesn't eat what I've prepared. "Nothing tastes the same."

"No" replaced "No thank-you" in 2020, and then became a simple shake of her head in 2021. Dementia continues to rob her of treasured vocabulary and me of her voice. A voice I long to hear, and to remember the sound of. There's grief in these losses prior to her physical death. The death of mother, the death of her voice, the death of me as daughter. And I'm sad. I watch and experience each day as I become more and more aware of the disease, the markers, next steps, and expected outcome. Mom is a beauty still, inside and out, as I write in 2021.

*What makes her Mom?* I contemplate as I record my grief. She's the mother I love, still physically present. However, the mom who loved her daughter, I mourn. Her shell, I love, but I miss my mom. So, I reflect.

Mom lived alone in Comox after retiring to the Comox Valley in 1998, just a few blocks away from our home, and her grandchildren. At the Seascape Apartments, she sought and found simplicity and security. An introvert, Mom found calm in her own company. Alone was her safe space. She lived alone ever since I headed to university in 1981, until moving into our home in January 2020.

Anytime Mom left her apartment, she'd be in a crisply pressed outfit. Her identity, she deemed, ready to be revealed. She didn't invite friends over or into her sanctuary, except on special occasions, at Thanksgiving or Christmas, when she made it ready. That space was hers alone.

"He was a well-to-do member of Vancouver society," she told me earlier when her mind was still sharp and focused, referring to my father. Then she'd clarified, as if it were important, "At least, his family was." Through the years, Mom shared sparse details, and only occasionally spoke of my dad. Theirs was a mysterious past she seemed reluctant to refresh in her mind's eye. But through the hazel eyes of this imaginative child, Mom's story was a real-life version of the classic Cinderella story, except with a dark twist after midnight.

She was invited on a date with a gallant officer, 2nd Lieutenant John Hall. He'd arrived in a chauffeur-driven Cadillac, dressed in a scarlet tunic, the uniform of an officer-in-training. He'd attended Royal Roads Military College, where affluent young men trained to be leaders.

"He pinned a corsage on the bodice of my gown," Mom said. He'd admired her beauty and gifted her an engraved silver bracelet, which she didn't want to accept. Her mother had told her when she was a young woman, "Sydney, it's inappropriate to accept expensive gifts from men." She only accepted after he pressed the Birks Jewellery box into her gloved hands and insisted. He encouraged her to open the gift-wrapped package with its trademark silver bow, and then to wear the engraved bracelet with her initials inscribed on her gloved wrist. Silver on white, her gloves were the expected formal wear and reached up past her elbows.

On dates, I imagined, my beautiful mother had attended lavish dinner parties. I later learned the Hall family had a gentleman's butler, maids, and hired help to polish silver. Tableware they used daily and to host luncheons included fine china, crystal, and a silver coffee and tea service. Seeing these fancy things at Christmas when Mom might bring out selected items, I'd ask, "What are all these things for?"

The Hall family regularly hosted dinner parties with friends, brokers at the stock exchange, assorted businessmen, and members of the Vancouver Board of Trade. I so easily pictured my mother as a Disney princess, dancing, losing track of time, and then suddenly surprised and horrified when the clock struck midnight and she found herself without her prince.

Mom, an elegant and charming new bride mastered the etiquette, and pretense required to belong. Who gave her the impression she wasn't enough? She seemed unaware when I was a child and later a teen of her identity beyond a mother. Her unique identity, masked at length, was lost during the masquerade. At a ball in 1957, she told me, my father, in military formal wear, had literally swept her off her feet, and asked her to marry. She fell into the arms of a man disguised as Prince Charming, it seemed. Sydney, in disguise as Cinderella, masked her identity cleverly.

Was it clever or fearfully that she masqueraded? Did she not know she was enough without a disguise? Was John, her suitor, masquerading as well? Why is it we wear masks so readily, fearing our authentic selves are not enough? Emily Swingler, Mom's mom, died of cancer at just fifty-four, in 1966. They'd both been smiling in 1960, when Mom had been a blushing bride. Was Grandma also unable to say, "Sydney, you are worthy, loved, and enough?" Had she died without her daughter being able to say, "I love you, Mom." Or hear, "I love you, Sydney" reciprocated?

"We received a hardware store as a wedding gift from the Hall family," Mom said. Upstairs was an apartment where the newlyweds settled. Despite Dad's parent's wealth, and his privileged upbringing, my father lacked prerequisite business acumen, according to Mom. Without initiative or independence, literally raised with silver service, he lacked the work ethic and aptitude to succeed in business or, more importantly, in relationships.

My courageous mom left my dad, she fled. She didn't want to carry on the masquerade. She was a beauty, inside and out, a genuine princess. I thought I knew her story as a child; however, I'd only imagined it. I would learn the truth, on a road trip, when there were just the two of us. With bravado, and uncharacteristic recklessness at fifteen, I asked as many pointed questions as the length of the trip and my daring allowed. She released few secrets from her vault.

I was just two in 1966, and my older sister, Sandra, was four, when my fierce warrior mama prioritized my sister and me and made a selfless choice. The story of my mother, for which I take full responsibility, is woven from these precious few gems, and a vivid imagination.

When was the beginning of Mom's inability to express herself verbally? She had difficulty saying no, and still does. Why? Was her inability to express herself prevalent when she was a child, or when she got married? Had she wanted something different from what her parents wanted for her and internalized her questions? Was it because her extroverted father, my grandpa, had said yes on her behalf without asking Mom if she'd wanted to model in a summer romper for a department store advertisement? Had her mother been distant and a difficult taskmaster? So many questions swirl and eddy in my mind. Did Emily, Mom's mom, verbalize her love? It's sad that I won't ever know, and hunger to understand. I speak and write "I love you" easily. These are words freely shared, sincerely from my thinly veiled heart. Yet, I'm easily wounded by silence. Unlike the palms of my hands, adapted for wear and tear, my heart is fragile, the pericardium a transparent veil, as I wait to hear Mom say, "I love you, Jocelyn."

JOCELYN BYSTROM

# CHAPTER EIGHT

**My Dad, The Stranger**

And what about my dad? Why did John Hall wait fifteen years to show up for me? I was seventeen when he arrived out of the blue. Arrived with nothing to say. All bottled up just like Mom. It appeared Dad, for all his problems with Mom, was just like her. He clearly wanted to connect, kept trying, but spontaneously, and without a plan. Each attempt left me confused and grieving, without an emotional repertoire to manage my wounds. Because he lacked fortitude and resilience to invest in our newly seeded relationship, each time I withered and died a little more.

He had forty-seven years to establish a relationship and spent as few as fourteen days reaching out to me. Was he ashamed? Was he bottled up for fifteen years, or drowning his sorrows in a bottle? Apologetic without an apology? Did I not deserve an explanation for his behaviour, or lack of action? Was he just another dad who couldn't bring himself to show up for life? His choices, whether he was aware or not, caused a lifetime of grief and mistrust. He left explanation to his abandoned child's imagination.

I wanted more.

~

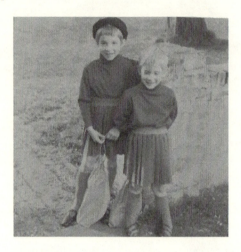

I'm on the right, with my older sister Sandra, ready for St. Christopher's private school, in Oak Bay, Victoria.

My parents moved from Vancouver to Kamloops, BC with their two infant girls. Shortly after my birth, my dad's aim was to operate the store they'd been gifted by his family. They settled upstairs in an apartment above their hardware store. Mom was busy with a new baby and my two-year-old sister, while Dad went downstairs to take care of business. Overwhelmed by the store's failure to thrive between 1964–1966, Dad self-medicated and, according to Mom, began hanging out with new friends at the hotel bar next door. "His new friends loved motorcycles," she said. Mom's tone and body language implied she did not.

~

Mom, in 1965, waited anxiously for her husband to come home each day. She worried every time Dad took Sandra, at three, then four, for rides on the back of his motorcycle. When I was a teen, selected stories emerged. "He became that husband and father who took my sister for rides while inebriated, and then lit the marital bed on fire after coming home drunk." She told me, "He'd been smoking in bed and passed out while his cigarette smouldered." The mattress, my mother disclosed from her vault of secrets, "needed to be thrown out the window, to keep the curtains and remaining furniture from catching fire." Thank goodness, I thought when she told me this, that she was awake and able to get rid of the burning mattress. Looking back, I'm grateful. The fire might have raged out of control while they slept. I too easily imagined catastrophic consequences.

Mom's fear of motorcycles became even more clear after my first few dates with Dale in 1982. Dale arrived on our front step, with his motorcycle helmet in hand, brown leather jacket, and mirrored sunglasses, after riding all the way back from a family reunion in BC, a nine-hour commute, to say "I missed you."

Mom looked out the picture window anxiously, hearing the roar of the engine, and then seeing someone coming up the path. While my heart leapt in anticipation of Dale's smiling blue eyes as he removed his sunglasses and helmet to give me a kiss, hers had lurched. Knowing he needed to win Mom's affection, and support for the question he'd returned home to ask, Dale had stopped to buy Mom flowers along the way. He'd already won my heart and soon I'd know the question he'd hurried home to ask. Without knowing a proposal was coming, "Yes" was already waiting on my lips.

~

The Hall family owned an entire apartment building and lived in the penthouse. They were investment bankers, I learned first from my mother at ten. Information which was then confirmed in 2020 when I found historical family memorabilia. Letters described my great-grandfather's travels from Minnesota to start a new bank in Winnipeg and then a brokerage firm in Vancouver, at the time a newly emerging city. Finding letters, detailed with memories, names, and dates, had become a necessary and appreciated lifeline.

In 2020, Mom's predictable answer to the question, "How are you, Sydney?" was "I don't want to say." Then after a pause, she'd add, "They've taken my brain away."

Grandpa Hall, Dad's dad, was a grandparent I have few memories of. I wasn't aware Mom had been in touch with Dad's parents until years later. Or that my dad apparently came to Courtenay, BC in June 1974, to sign divorce papers. Papers I read for the first time in 2021 which said, "This court doth decree and adjudge that the petitioner, John Franklin Hall, pay the respondent, Sydney Carol Hall, the sum of one dollar ($1.00 CAD) per year, beginning on the 1st day of July 1974, and thereafter a like sum of one dollar ($1.00) on the first day of July in every succeeding year."

No, it's not a mistake. One dollar to support "the infant children was to be paid." This after my dad had failed to pay the arrears totalling $3,200 CAD from a 1967 judgement, which was later reduced in 1974, to $1,100 CAD. He was given permission to pay the lesser amount in installments of twenty-five dollars a month beginning in July 1974. This when a quart of milk cost $1.39 and a gallon of gas would have cost my mom fifty-three cents to drive to work, to take us to highland dancing lessons or my sister to gymnastics. Dad sent nothing; he said nothing.

Mom communicated with my dad periodically about our welfare and successes in school, although my sister and I were unaware. You can imagine my shock when he showed up unexpectedly at my high school graduation.

"Hi Jocelyn, I'm your dad." I certainly wouldn't have known he was my father except that he'd just stated it. This, as he walked up to me in the school hallway where I was lined up to have a graduation portrait taken, excitedly chatting with friends. He had called earlier to say he might be coming. *Why?* I didn't really think he would. He was my father, but there was no love shared or seeds of nurture taking root. Who was this man claiming, "I'm your dad"?

Mom's bottled up for one reason; Dad is bottled up for another. Both bottles were being poured into my cup, which was still empty. They didn't provide me with the tools I needed to navigate challenges met throughout childhood and adolescence, or the mental health "earthquake" at fifty, when the earth shifted unexpectedly beneath my feet.

Dad had many opportunities to reach out before my high school graduation, and then again for nearly three decades after. In fact, he had forty-four years, or sixteen thousand and sixty opportunities, to pick up a phone or write a letter and sign it *Love, Dad*.

There were brief, halting phone calls, and short visits when I hadn't known what to do with my hands except fidget, as thoughts and questions spiralled in my busy brain. There was the call at seventeen two days prior to graduation, another at eighteen, while I was in my first year of university, and later an unexpected invitation, which left me flummoxed. A strange pattern emerged where my dad would call, saying, "Hi, it's your dad...." Calls which left me wounded and baffled, questioning his intent.

In 1982, he asked if I would come to Vancouver. He was getting remarried. With seconds to consider this bizarre request, there came another, a real doozy. "I want you to take part in the bridal party, as the maid of honour." He didn't even ask. He just stated his needs.

Wasn't the maid of honour chosen by the bride? I'd questioned. He wanted me to fly from Edmonton, Alberta to Vancouver, British Columbia, for a wedding of two people I barely knew.

"Is Sandra invited?" I asked, bewildered. Had he forgotten he had two children? I wouldn't go without her.

Ultimately, we went, because I'm a pleaser. I still had residual hope for a father/daughter relationship. I'm an eternal optimist. The wedding itself was all too weird and easily buried. From the moment we arrived till we left I felt like a performer in an elaborate charade. Did Dad even know the colour of my eyes? Guests most likely had more questions than polite courtesy allowed them to ask. Why was the maid of honour the groom's daughter? With our forgettable performance over, Sandra and I fled to the airport, the wedding easily forgotten in the rear view mirror.

A month after the wedding, Dad phoned again. "I think we're trying to bridge an ungappable bridge. I'm sorry." Then he hung up. What he meant, although leaving me bewildered was that he'd tried, but couldn't do it. The bridge he was trying to cross back to me had been blown to smithereens.

He made it easier, a lot easier, not to send a wedding invite when I got married to Dale the following year. We wouldn't communicate again for another eleven years. Not until after I became a mother. Maybe, I thought, he'd want to know I was a parent, and that he was a grandpa. This time, I called.

"Thank you for letting me know," was all he said.

At forty-five, I finished my master's degree, and earned my position as a gifted education specialist, teaching Challenge. I was flourishing, proud of the home Dale and I had created for our family, and excited about possibilities. Mom was well-established, after her retirement from teaching, and living in the Comox Valley. Now, she was a devoted, beloved grandparent. Dad called again. He'd had a series of strokes, and recently a big one. His second wife had died, and he was in hospital. He needed me.

Initially, I hadn't realized it was even my dad because the stroke had left his speech significantly impaired. I thought it was a crank call, that the person phoning was drunk, and I almost hung up. Again, he wanted me to travel to Vancouver, a five-hour trip, to visit him in hospital. A trip which would require an overnight stay in the Vancouver area. An excursion which included a ferry crossing the Georgia Strait, arranging time off, and ensuring my responsibilities at home and work would be covered. Uncertain, I asked Dale if I should go.

"He is your dad, and family," he replied. So, we went. A child, ever ready to please.

Thankfully, Dale accompanied me to Vancouver General Hospital. I needed his strength to manage the visit. There, I struggled to explain to the ICU nurse why my dad, who couldn't clearly speak after his life-threatening stroke, was crying. She couldn't quite grasp that a daughter didn't know which of the four men in the room was her father, or how he wouldn't immediately recognize me either. Somehow, he had known. I hadn't. It was hard, and my chest felt ready to implode. Words didn't flow, although he tried, but couldn't. Eventually, the nurse gave him paper and pen. He wrote, *Sorry*.

A year later came another call. Knowing, yet not sharing that he was terminally ill, he pleaded, "Please, Jocelyn, can I come and visit you over the Christmas holidays?"

I was quiet just a little too long. A pregnant pause, which felt otherworldly. Somehow, I sensed it was his dying wish. It was the right thing to do. He needed me. I felt nudged. *He's family*, I heard my inner child and Dale reiterate. It wasn't about me. Each time Dad connected, my heart would hope, and the girl in the mirror waited in expectation to hear, "*I love you, Jocelyn.*" It didn't occur to me then that my dad was the needy child, or that I had become his caregiver.

Hesitantly, I said yes.

That Christmas, during his two-week visit, when I wasn't caregiving—feeding the family or arranging for his care—I lay on our couch and feigned sleep. Who was this old man in my living room? Why was he here? What was I supposed to say? I closed my eyes to not have to acknowledge his presence while he sat staring at me. Neither of us had words. I didn't know our days and months were numbered.

My mind raced with anxiety that Christmas as I struggled to understand what went through my dad's mind the day, he had arrived home in 1966 to an empty apartment, or any day thereafter. He wasn't around to ask.

I didn't know from year to year if he was alive, dead, or disinterested. Were we a burden? Why didn't he care enough to keep in touch, express his feelings, or visit? Do you earn the right to be called Dad, or simply attain it? I didn't have a dad who chose to be present, express affection, or attempt to communicate, until *he* decided it was time. I was caught in the middle of two troubled bookends who could neither express themselves nor offer the needed answers.

On Feb.6, 2010, Dad died on my birthday.

# CHAPTER NINE

### Bossy Jocie

I'm four. It's September 1968. I'm too young to be at school, but Mom is a single parent, so I go to pre-kindergarten at St. Christopher's private school, where I'm told I am to wear a uniform. I must. Sandra and I both must, and we do as we're told. I don't know why, but sometimes the teacher calls me Jocie. Doesn't she know my name is Jocelyn? One day, we're singing, and the teacher asks us to think of words that rhyme with our names. Mine's hard to rhyme, and I can't think of one. Then one kid suggests "Bossy Jocie." I don't like that. I'm not bossy. All the kids laugh at me. What does it mean to be bossy, anyway?

Sandra and I go to school in black or brown saddle shoes, grey knee socks, and a grey pleated skirt with an elastic waistband. There's one choice, a blue blouse or blue turtleneck, dependent on the season. All the kids must wear a grey tam-o'-shanter on our heads, which is a flat, round bonnet, usually made of felted wool with a pompom ; it's part of our uniform. I hate hats. I'm always pulling off my tam and getting into trouble.

One morning, I hide under a group of desks and wait in silence. It's a game, and I'm excited with tingles. I wonder if anyone will notice my safe hiding place? Sandra usually finds the best spots when we play hide-and-seek, but not today. I'm uncertain how long I'm there, but it seems exceptionally long.

Longer than I wanted the game to last. I smile when I hear them looking for me. It's my turn to have the best hiding spot. Adults rush around. I'm good at being quiet. Won't they be surprised when they discover my wonderful hiding place. I'm a mouse, not moving my whiskers, just my eyes, listening.

I wait too long. No one seems happy anymore. In fact, there's one lady standing so close I can't see her from between the legs of the desks but imagine as I listen that her chest is puffed out, the veins on her neck are bulging, and that her shoulders are up by her ears. Then suddenly all her breath escapes and she made a weird noise, like "Huuhh." Next, I hear heels tapping on the floor, as another person comes close. I can only see their legs and feet as they stand talking. Their voices sound shaky and loud, and they rush off, asking, "Has anyone seen Jocelyn?"

*Is something wrong?*

My four-year-old mind doesn't understand. I slip out and pretend the game is over. I don't understand why I get in trouble. They must have wanted to find my special, secret hiding place. I don't tell them about it because they forgot to ask. Then I hear that lady with the choppy voice. I think she's the headmistress. She's talking on the phone. "She's been found," she says. They must have found someone else's hiding spot; they didn't find mine.

It's Saturday and I'm turning five.

Monday morning, we go to our new school called Monterey Elementary, and I start grade one. There, girls must wear dresses. Only boys get to wear long pants. I miss my old primary school where we used to write notes home to our moms on pretty paper before we went on field trips. Once, my teacher asked the class to copy a letter to parents from the blackboard:

*Dear Mom,*
*I must be spic and span and span and spic for my field trip to*

*the Crystal Gardens Swimming Pool next week. I need to bring my bathing suit.*
   *Love, Jocelyn*

I write "Love," just like my mom writes it on my birthday card. The other kids copy the teacher's letter correctly. I was supposed to write "From Jocelyn."

One morning, it's just my sister and me. We are home alone and waiting for the correct time to leave for school. It's just minutes since our babysitter left to go to her school. Sandra, seven now and in grade two, is to remember what time we are supposed to leave. While we wait, we decide to make paper chains because it's almost Christmas and we want to decorate our house. We cut long strips of red and green because everyone knows these are the Christmas colors. Sandra wrinkles up her nose and face and I see she's remembered to read the clock on the stove. We've made a lovely long chain that stretches all the way across the kitchen and into the living room. Mom's going to love it. Except, Sandra says, "We're late, really late for school."

We look at each other, wondering what to do. We're well-behaved, never late. "What do we do?" I ask my big sister, feeling like I have marbles in my stomach. "I don't want to go."

"I want to go to school," Sandra insists. "Mom will find out if we don't."

I know what happens to children in my class who are late for school and stand my ground. "I'm not going." But she's older, and in charge, and getting ready to leave. And more than I don't want to go, I don't want to be left alone.

Arriving at school, I wish I could hide. An adult passing us in the hallway tells us, "You need to go to the office and get a late slip." I know about the office. It's a place where bad boys go. I know this because a boy in my class who lied to the teacher made her mad. She told him in a loud voice, like the police officer directing traffic at an intersection, "Go to the office."

I make my sister go in first while I hide around the

corner. "Will you get me one?" I whisper. But she's already gone in and doesn't hear, which means I must follow her into that place. I get the shivers, even though I'm still wearing my coat. Then I remember Mom's cautionary reminder. I must take off the pants I'm wearing under my dress, because girls aren't allowed to wear pants. I don't want to get caught even though they're great pants for climbing trees, stretchy with blue and white zigzags.

I choose my own clothes now, which I like. Sandra chooses clothes that match, not me. I like bright colours, and whatever calls to me when I open the drawer. I take off my favourite jazzy pants, as Mom calls them. Mom will be proud of me because I've remembered.

"Sandra and Jocelyn Hall . . . Late - 9:48 a.m.," the lady with the glasses behind the desk says as she writes our names in a big binder then gives us each a small paper with only the word "LATE" on it. We must give the slip to our teachers. As Sandra walks me to class, I think about what my teacher will say, and the other kids will think. Mrs. Talbot might not like me anymore.

My sister drops my hand, leaving me standing outside my closed classroom door, and heads off. She seems like she wants to get to class quickly. I'm all alone and dreading turning the handle to go in. I'm still there when the teacher notices me.

"Come in, Jocelyn," she says, speaking in the same tone my mother used when we climb up high in the maple tree. She tells me I must stay after school and clean the blackboard brushes. It can't be my punishment for being late, I think. I love to clean the blackboard brushes and have volunteered to stay before to do it. Helping makes me feel special. I'm good at it. All day I wonder, what will my punishment be?

I don't need a babysitter anymore, I tell my teacher after school, when she asks who is picking me up today.

I get my lunch kit and book bag ready. "My sister's waiting for me," I say. "May I go?" She replies, "You may." I open the classroom door and close it behind me. My big sister is there, waiting for me. We live just down the street from our school, so we walk home together and then play in our backyard till Mom gets home from work.

Sandra and I like to climb up into the gigantic maple tree in our backyard. It's fantastic to climb with its strong, reaching branches. Once, my mom looked out our second-story window and spotted us. We were higher than her.

"Come down right away!" she said in a sharp voice she rarely uses, then added, "Be careful! Hold on tight." Her eyes were dark and full of fear. Perhaps she didn't know what good climbers we were. But we climbed down anyway.

Just before Valentine's Day on my sixth birthday, I receive a package with my name on it. "It's not from me," Mom says. I'm not sure who it's from, but it doesn't matter, because it's for me. It's a yellow dump truck. I make mud pies in the backyard and love that gift. It wasn't like any present Mom gave me. Could it be from my dad? I hoped so. Maybe he hasn't forgotten me.

At seven, I find a photograph of mom in a white, fur-trimmed figure skating dress.

"It's mine," I tell my sister. I want control, too, and don't seem to have any. My things become precious treasures. I don't always want to share, just because we're sisters. Mom's photograph is framed behind gold etched glass. I love touching its soft brown velvet backing while I gaze at her. The girl in the photograph—Mom yet not the mom I know—seems so mysterious.

I once got into trouble for reaching out and touching a tall lady's coat at Woodward's department store as we rode up on the escalator. We were headed from ladies' fashions on the first floor to the children's department on the second. I hoped we might shop for new winter jackets. My old one, soft like my teddy bear, with its fluffy hood trimmed with white fur, was getting too small. Mom told me it was fake fur, but I loved it anyway. I watched my feet as we went up, up, up. I was mesmerized. Then I noticed someone in front of me wearing a long, dreamy winter coat just one step away, so close I could reach out and touch it. So, I did. This must be what real fur feels like, I thought. She must be very rich. I wanted one.

My fingers caressed and lingered in the softness, until my mother noticed and was horrified. Like lightening she reached down and swept my offending hand away. She then clasped my hand and gave me a look that spoke volumes without words. As I looked up, I saw her furrowed brow and *I can't believe you just did that* look. The look, where Mom tilts her head and raises her eyebrows. Apparently, fancy ladies on escalators don't appreciate small children pawing expensive fur coats. At home later, Mom said, "That was real fur, and very expensive. You must not touch."

But I was careful, I thought.

Mom is always saying, "Be careful." Is this her cautionary way of telling me to expect bad things if I touch? Is she suggesting I'm not capable of disguising my touch, or to manage without her? She's wrong. I can handle it. I did. Had that lady even noticed? I didn't think so. My fingers are like whispers. No one even notices me.

I have so many questions about that photograph of Mom in her figure skating dress. I lay on my bed and imagine possibilities. I fantasize about my mother. That girl in the photograph is begging to tell her story. My mother doesn't tell me. Is her story a secret?

The mom, I imagine, differs from the mom who comes home from work at the hospital. Hospital mom has her white lab coat on. I prefer the mom in her beautiful, white fur-trimmed skating dress. Fur-trimmed mom, I imagine, would always smile, and reach for my hand lovingly. She would be a mom with energy to cuddle after a twelve-hour shift and time for bedtime stories. She might be like Dick and Jane's mom, who read stories, and stayed at home with her children, while Father went to work. I'm smart though and know those moms aren't real. They're only in storybooks. I read about those imaginary moms in my reader at school. Not every family has a dad, a mom that stays home, or a dog named Spot, at least not in my family.

Real moms love you but go to work. They are busy and tired when they get home. My mom needs to take care of the house, make supper, do the dishes, and pack school lunches for tomorrow. I knew my mom loved us. She would write *Love, Mom* on my birthday card. She was a single parent and worked extremely hard to take care of us. But she wasn't home much.

When Mom got home, she was tired, got quiet, and I often wondered why. Did she need someone to take care of her?

Except on Sundays, which were Mom's day off. Then she had time and a slight smile. After church, we would go to Cadboro Bay Park to play. This was my mom. My mom got me ready for the lady, the sitter, or someone she trusted to come and stay with us. People who came before school, after school, or to tuck us in when Mom worked late. Sometimes our sitter, an older lady, would be the one to say goodnight.

"Mom's at work, dear. She'll be home soon."

That lady doesn't come anymore. I'm almost eight. Sandra's in charge. We manage just fine. My mom, the girl behind the glass in my photograph, who is poised and confident in her skating dress, what happened to that girl? That girl in her blue velvet, fur-trimmed dress ready to perform her solo on ice skates. Where is her mom? Mom doesn't seem to manage without her.

My mom, the mom who tucks me in, when possible, is a lady who might stand at the edge of a crowded room, observant and watchful. I imagine her at parents' night at my school, while we were at home with a sitter. She'd be the well-dressed quiet lady, scanning the room. Attending because it's expected and the right thing to do. Mom always meets her obligations. Tonight, she might be seated and waiting. She'll be contemplating the just right time it's socially acceptable to give herself permission to escape. She's ready to be home with her girls, pay our sitter, and get some sleep.

Mom's busy brain is always thinking and ready to run.

While other parents huddle and chat socially, waiting for the meeting to begin, I imagine Mom planning her disappearance into the fog, just like the ferry I saw leaving for Port Angeles. She will slip away, while others engage in conversation unaware, hoping to leave without being judged for prioritizing her girls. She'll slip away like last time, on the train, while Dad was at work unsuspecting. Before anyone gets close, Mom will excuse herself, in a voice barely above a whisper, "I'm sorry, I need to go...to get home to my girls." Appearances and etiquette matter.

We had the book *Miss Manners' Book of Etiquette* on the shelf beside the dining room table. Mom brought it home. She wants us to be well-mannered and reminds us not to slurp through the straw, or drink juice from the jug. Mom would be the last mother to wear curlers in public or leave the house without a coordinating lipstick and handbag. We must not accidentally use the dinner fork instead of the proper salad fork to eat the side salad. When I investigate the fancy wooden chest on top of the buffet hutch, I notice forks that look like spoons, and ask, "What are these?"

"They're dessert forks—half spoon, half fork—to eat ice cream and cake." Then Mom adds, "They go to the right of the knife and teaspoon on the right." Apparently, a dessert fork is necessary, so I don't lick the last of the velvety, melted ice-cream off my plate. Heaven forbids.

"There once was a girl, who had a little curl, right in the middle of her forehead. When she was good, she was very, very good, but when she was bad, she was naughty." That's the way I remember Mom reciting the verse. I only lick the plate when Mom isn't watching, since I'm a good girl. A good girl with a naughty streak, and I'm pretty sure each time mom reads or recites the verse from our book of rhymes, it's about me. I am that girl. The one with the curl.

"No way, not my mom." She had curls but was never naughty. She'd feel naked without lipstick and naked she would never be. Not my mother. I wonder in passing if behind closed doors she ever likes to run, jump, or play hide-and-seek? Does she ever let down her long, blond hair with its natural curls? I loved those curls and wanted my own.

"Please pin-curl my hair tonight?" I'd ask every night with pins in hand.

She always said yes. I wonder why she doesn't say no very often. I try not to take advantage of mom's inability to say no most days. Sometimes I know she's too tired to curl my hair, but I still want curls. I appreciate the yes. Maybe she didn't hear yes much when she asked questions? Did she ask as many questions as I do? Probably not.

Today, Mom keeps her hair short. Is it because it's easy to take care of? It was a similar style to what we had when we were younger, the "pixie cut." A style my sister and I have hated since that day at the park when we were playing on the slide. Some mean boys stared at us and said, "Boys don't wear dresses. Why are you wearing dresses?" Mom heard what they said. Sandra and I decided on the spot to grow our hair long. We're girls. Why are boys so mean? Maybe I shouldn't ask so many questions. I sure wish Mom would tell me what it was like when she was a little girl. Was she like me?

Mom is a master at changing the subject. Her thoughts are hers alone. I, too, guard my thoughts. Mom talks about us, not herself. She talks about "her girls," not her past, and then asks, "Where might you like to move next?"

"Somewhere with snow" was our simultaneous, jubilant plea. I wondered later whether it had been a duet, or simply my big sister's answer? Did I simply remember it as ours? Had I simply answered inside my head. That voice is very loud. Sometimes I don't know if I've spoken out loud or not.

That winter, we go exploring. We get into our Austin mini and drive north from Victoria, British Columbia, where we live in Oak Bay. Are we headed to find snow? I hope so. It turns out that we are, and we do. We drive all the way to Courtenay, and drive up the mountain, following the signs with skiers on them to Forbidden Plateau. Mom says we'll find snow there. We sing on the way as Mom drives. Between songs, while it's quiet, I think. Mom will be proud of me because I've learned to keep my thoughts in my head just like her. I decide I already know her answer about letting her hair down, the answer to the question I'd been thinking about when I wondered: Did Mom ever play, or ask silly questions? The answers I'm sure of now and hear in my head. No, and no.

Did we find snow? We did, and a year later, we moved to the Comox Valley. We moved to Courtenay and 728-8th Avenue across the lane from what would be our new school. All, I believed, because we'd found snow at Forbidden Plateau. Was that really the reason we moved there, or only what I naively believed? What a curious name for a ski hill. Such great snow.

In the early 1970s, after moving to Courtenay, north of Victoria on Vancouver Island, I learn my grandparents, Dad's parents, took responsibility for us, when my dad had not. They set up a trust fund for each of us, my sister and me. A trust which paid out one hundred dollars each month into an account saved for our care. Grandpa Hall also set up a small trust to pay for university when we turned eighteen. Mom needed to use "our money," as she called it, sometimes. Each time, she'd apologize.

"I'm so sorry, girls. I need to dip into the money from Grandpa Hall this month."

Later, when I was older, I would often say, "Mom, it's okay. You don't need to apologize." She often apologized for things that were no fault of hers, and I'd need to remind her.

Why she carried such guilt, I've never understood. She was intelligent and well educated. She worked long hours first as a dietician in hospitals, and then taking additional training while teaching full time to become a home economics teacher. We'd returned with her to the University of British Columbia over several summers while she completed her teacher's training. Mom was not a slacker. She was industrious, capable, and provided for us to the best of her ability. I never felt we lacked for anything—except hugs and words of affection.

JOCELYN BYSTROM

# CHAPTER TEN

### A Feel Good Place

Where would my feet land and stick? Where might tender roots become established and find a forever home? We moved to the Comox Valley, north of Victoria on Vancouver Island, where there would be another new bedroom, lunch kit, and classroom full of taller kids. We moved and then moved again from one home to the next. My sister and I attended a new school each year. We were always on the move. I was constantly seeking that one, someone special, to call a friend. I hoped to establish lasting friendships beyond June. Only to learn, once again, I'd have another penfriend.

Mom allowed us to get a pet, much to our delight. Tippee, our mutt with the spotted tail, grew much bigger than the man at the SPCA promised. We were busy, mom was at work, and our lonely dog barked, which annoyed the neighbors. Sadly, he was returned to the pound. We were those people. We got a calico kitten. Cats, Mom hoped, would be more independent. Our dog, the sweet calico cat, who had six kittens, and then a hamster—no pet lasted, or was around long enough to be captured in a treasured scrapbook.

In the early 1970s, Sandra and I sang along with the car radio on our way to pick up Mom's colleague from work, Carole. "I'd like to buy the world a Coke and keep it company. I'd like to teach the world to sing in perfect harmony…"

We joined in and belted out The Coca-Cola Company's jingle, the lyrics to one of my favourite songs about apple trees and honeybees, as we headed with Carole to Bates Beach. Mom said we could learn to fish. We're west coasters now, and we learned to do all the things that people who live here liked to do. We learned about Northern Coast Salish peoples who lived here thousands of years ago in this Land of Plenty.

Who wears a purple muumuu to go fishing? Carole does. Carole, like us, had never been fishing. The man at the boat launch, Mr. Bates, taught Mom to operate the outboard motor and use the fishing rod. He said something about trolling for salmon. With a pull, he started the motor for us. With a push, he launched us from shore, and we were off. My fearless, intrepid mom operated the outboard motor. With one hand she held the tiller secure with fingers like the jaws on a pair of vice-grips, while her other secured her fear to the rail. She steered us in the direction Mr. Bates had pointed towards the other boats, which appeared to be going back and forth in a long, slow pattern. Mom had that telling look on her face. Her skin was all pinched and her eyes were squinty while she focused on the task at hand. Carole, in her purple muumuu, was oblivious and took photographs.

Mom got the rod in the water, and we fished, sort of. Then, Mom saw her boss, the principal from her school where she worked. He looked over at us, smiled, and waved. Mom didn't seem too pleased to see him and gave him one of those smiles with her lips pursed together and the skin pulled tight across her face. Unlike her other smile when her blue eyes sparkle, lines crease from the corners of her eyes and her teeth peek from between Maybelline or Revlon coloured lips. Mom steered our boat away and we headed sight-seeing instead. It was no surprise we didn't catch any fish, looking back.

I did, however, catch a deep appreciation for my mother, who seemed willing to try most anything, even when it was hard. Next up, we learned to ski. Her girls, as she called us, must not miss out. I loved this place and had secured a best friend, Amy, who had five siblings, and a mom who didn't mind that her daughter spent almost all her time with me. Amy's mom would say, "You girls are just like two peas in a pod." We'd moved into a big house in Courtenay, near Puntledge Park, and I had my very own room. We didn't share our house with another family, it was just ours. I wanted to stay, but we didn't.

I was never sure why.

In the Comox Valley, between 1971–1974, Sandra and I learned to fish, ski, and highland dance. And at school we learned about the indigenous peoples, known as the K'ómoks First Nation, who used cedar roots to build watertight cooking baskets and pots, and large cedars for totem poles and beams for their Big Houses. I could be at home here among the tall cedars, deer, elk, and eagles, I thought. I loved to swim in the Puntledge River, and to go to the beach. Everywhere it seemed the forest and mountains touched the sky and to this day the indigenous peoples speak of the legend of Queneesh. A legend, which speaks of a white whale stranded high on the mountain near PE'ntlatc Lake, a legend which suggests that when the water froze, the whale could not get away. Still frozen, it can be seen there to this day, as the Comox Valley glacier, called Queneesh.

Like Canada geese we leave the valley of Queneesh and migrate to another place. Flying east to I know not where. We move to another new place. Where we're going, I'm unaware. We pack our things, and I say a prayer.

Will it be a feel-good place, or an I want to leave place? What is it about a place that makes Mom want to be there or to flee? Am I the only one who wants to stay? It felt like home to me.

~

It would take another twelve years to find my feel-good place. In a loving, committed relationship, I landed on solid ground, when at nineteen, Dale asked me to marry. In marriage and in each other's arms, I found home.

Commitment, I believed, and vowing "until death do us part" promised me I could safely tear down the walls I had built around my heart. Dale would be my forever home, I promised myself. I would experience a sense of deep connection and rootedness in us. Our home would always have a foundation of love.

Dale and I landed in the Comox Valley, after our first years together and committed to establishing roots in our new community, friendships, the neighbourhood, and, after baptising our firstborn, at church.

Home was where we brought our babies from the hospital, just two blocks from where each of our children were born. Here, two adoring grandmas, one Nana, the other Grandma, welcomed our newborns. Our home became a place of peace and sanctuary, and later a place our adult children returned to visit, much to our delight.

Through the years, Mom would visit our home frequently, almost daily, after she moved to the Comox Valley. There were a few extended stays with us through the years when she'd needed our support. When the COVID-19 pandemic threatened, Mom moved in for what we believed would be another short stay to keep her safe during the pandemic.

My sanctuary, home and heart, experienced a significant shift when Mom moved in. Where did her needs end and mine begin? New unexpected responsibilities arrived alongside her diagnosis with frontal temporal dementia. I became a full-time caregiver.

I finalized Mom's tenancy at the Seascape Apartments over the next few months. Unbeknownst to her, I turned the key and engaged the deadbolt on a now emptied apartment.

As someone who cherishes family, it was easy to say yes, and have Mom stay. I framed photographs and hung memorabilia as I decorated her new room. She seemed pleased to be there, without mention of what was, had been, or knowledge of what she previously may have missed or grieved leaving behind. Forgotten were her belongings, memories made, as she began living in the present with increasingly fewer words and memories.

I was inspired to write. Sitting to collect my thoughts I began to record what she and I remembered. The collage of words, phrases, and photos captured the essence of all the most important relationships in my life. Each paragraph detailed a beautiful human I gave thanks for, prayed for, or delighted in, as my own mental, spiritual, emotional, and physical health declined.

No longer was I that little girl who laughed and giggled with delight when Grandpa Swingler visited. My favorite grandpa, who I loved immeasurably and who had joined us for cartwheel races in our backyard, died in 1978, when I was fourteen. I hadn't realized yet what I would miss most. My beloved Grandpa had known how to bring me out of my shell when I felt shy or needed a pep talk. I needed my grandpa, now, after my integrity and professionalism were called into question and my confidence shattered. Grief spoke volumes in 2020, as I sat and mourned suppressed losses ready to erupt.

Thoughts percolated as if from a volcanic vent after I'd made humiliating mistakes in 2014 and was told my apology wasn't sincere or acceptable. Grandpa would have known what to say. How to make me smile again. It was then I became even more accomplished at masking fear and burying pain.

*Grandpa, where were the people like you, who believed in me, and would stand up for me, when untruths were being told.* Their silence spoke volumes.

*Grandpa, I need you now.*

I lift my fingers and caress an earring now and remember. You're here with me even now, Grandpa. Year after year on my birthday there'd be a blue velvet box from Birks Jewellery, and inside the iconic Birks blue, amethyst jewelry for my February birthday.

I learned early to build walls masterfully and control

appearances. Silently, and in pain, I mourned the loss of his unconditional love and support. Fitting in a pair of amethyst earrings gifted to me at thirteen, I wear a brave mask at fifty.

Each gift received from Grandpa was given from his heart to mine, rather than to purchase my affection. I felt it in the warmth of his words and sheltering hugs, and as I watched him cartwheel in our backyard.

Closing my eyes again, right in front of me, I see and remember the turquoise, velvet box. One each Christmas, each birthday, and always inside each lid his curvy handwriting ensuring I'd always know...

*Love Always, Grandpa.*

I was your jewel, and still, he can make me sparkle. You're at home, in my heart, Grandpa.

*Grandpa, is home inside me?*

~

Family is home now. Our home, where we hope and I'm prayerful that our children and their partners, and perhaps grandchildren, will continue to visit and return. Home is where we work diligently side by side with a consistent shared vision.

Our adult son, Keith, visited and gifted me freshly painted walls in my new home office. Pale green walls created calm in 2020. Keith visited, observed, and listened to my heart, then applied semi-gloss after I'd imagined a home office. A nurturing, feel-good space where I could sit to create.

He brought the serenity of the forest inside, at a time when I was struggling and needed structure and routine. There also just happened to be a worldwide pandemic. Now I could enjoy a peaceful place to sit and write.

Unbeknownst to me, Dale would become my caregiver and care-partner, in addition to my best friend, within the next six months. Mom and I would suddenly share much more than a roof over our heads. The unimaginable happened at the end of January 2020, when within two days of each other, we'd both experienced the loss of our driver's licences. Within six months, loved ones would observe significant cognitive decline in both mother and daughter. Home, without warning, would feel like a prison without an ability to escape or the possibility of parole. I was all in.

I lost myself at home, amidst the pandemic, in the deep recesses of my mind and body. My new feel-good place would be outside under our covered deck, seated and tucked beneath a cozy quilt lovingly handmade by a treasured friend, with a hot cup of tea. There I found temporary reprieve, escape, and a home away from home. Just me, alone with my thoughts. Sometimes it was a scary place to call home. Why was I so desperate to leave this place? What was it about being at home, in my head and heart, that made me want to flee?

~

I created a collage of family photographs—a "Wall of Love"—that embraced my heart as I sat to write of struggles, challenges, and losses. I was held. Beautiful humans I gave thanks for, prayed for, who delighted in me, believed in me and who were present witnessing my decline.

No longer was I that little girl, who laughed and giggled with delight when Grandpa Swingler visited. Now, I was in pain—deep pain over loss secreted away and unresolved grief. My favorite grandpa, who I'd loved immeasurably, was only a distant memory. Grandpa, who'd known just how to bring me out of my interior life, was one of very few. He saw deeper and took the time to ask and listen. My grandpa didn't judge or make assumptions based solely on my actions or appearance. He observed with his heart and saw the shy, little girl, lacking confidence with woolen ribbons tied in her pencil-thin pigtails.

My honesty, integrity, and professionalism were called into question in 2014. I once was and am again wounded, alone, silenced, and fearful. I believed others, who knew me as Grandpa did, would have my back. But by their silence, I was convicted.

I assumed naively, once again that little girl, that they'd cared. Don't they see me, know me, or care? I'd wondered. They said my apology was "unacceptable" and "I'm insincere and highly unprofessional."

Any compliments, encouragement, and kind words I've received, earned, and heard vanished as if never uttered. Instead, my brain clung to the insults, criticism, and judgement. Years later, I still relive hearing, seeing, and finding myself stepping back into this scene. Over and over and over I hear: "unacceptable, insincere, and highly unprofessional." Roles are reversed. I'm the antagonist unable of letting go of this new script, which battles endlessly on automatic replay. I have a starring role in a horror movie that I didn't audition for, but find myself cast in, nonetheless.

When my honesty, integrity and professionalism were called into question, my response had been to silence myself again. My reaction to the email I'd written after my career-ending job loss felt like a gag order. Although self-imposed, I believed speaking up for myself was taboo. Even then, I'd been accomplished at masking fear and burying trauma. I'd learned early to masterfully build walls and control appearances for self-protection. It had been a self-preservation tactic, one I would return to again and again when triggered.

Insults injure and words re-traumatize. I'm deserving, I'm told, of reprimand. I hear and internalize this harsh reality. I deserve this. Do I deserve this? I do. Do I? I don't think so.

With my thoughts, I battle. I fight for my interior life, believing I'm a good person, and have integrity. I pressed send; It's true. I'm responsible for my actions. Also, true. Did I intend others harm? Absolutely not. Did I harm anyone? Had I meant to? Perhaps, I did. Perhaps I wanted retaliation after anger percolated. I *was* hurt and wounded. I *was* angry and lashed out. Am I proud of this realization? No. The indirect result of this misdeed was that I won't ever win the battle. I constantly duel without weapons, silenced by shame. In choosing silence there are ripples.

I was accomplished at masking fear and burying sadness and pain. I'd learned early to masterfully build barricades and control outward appearances. No one, I vowed, would see me cry, as I left the disciplinary meeting.

~

It had taken years to find my feel-good place. In a loving, committed relationship called marriage, and in Dale's arms, I'd found home. Being loved unconditionally had allowed me to start tearing down walls in a relationship where my heart knew safety. At home I could speak my truth, experience my feelings whatever they may be, and express myself authentically in a reciprocal trusting relationship.

Deep roots were created after thirty-four years of marriage. Our home was a love nest we built together and a place of connection and safety. Until all that changed.

JOCELYN BYSTROM

# PART THREE

## SEASON OF WAITING

JOCELYN BYSTROM

# CHAPTER ELEVEN

### Who Holds Your Hand?

Between 2014–2020, while waiting for clarity following each diagnostic test, my physical health declined. Unacknowledged emotions breathed energy into my fears, and I became fixated on physical challenges I anticipated moving forward. Would I be able to walk at sixty, or need a rolling walker as the neurologist had suggested? Would I have the energy to do the things I loved: walk and run in the Northeast woods, snowshoe up Mt. Washington, or swim across Sproat Lake? Would I be able to offer support to my children when they became parents, to confidently hold a grandchild securely? Who would take over the responsibility of caring for Mom when she needed a ride to her favourite park or to go to church? Who would hold Dale's hand, if not me?

I became overwhelmed with apprehension about a future of caregiving, and unable to enjoy a present or future I'd assumed would be mine. Unrealistic expectations of what I needed to manage swirled and spiralled out of control.

Being chosen as Mom's power of attorney (POA) had been an honour that I accepted with ease. When my intelligent brain was still fully functioning, Mom and I sat together at the kitchen table, reviewing an advanced care planning document titled *My Voice, Expressing My Wishes for Future Health Care Treatment*. I'd printed two blank copies and we filled them out side by side. I thought this would be easier for Mom, telling her that it was something everyone needed to do, me included. I knew this to be true, and believed it wholeheartedly, but at the time thought it a clever ploy to initiate a potentially difficult conversation. In fact, I hadn't realized I would also need to choose a POA and complete these same forms so soon.

What was a manageable level of responsibility as Mom's POA in 2018 shifted into more of a full-time job by 2020. My role morphed slowly from daughter to care-partner, twenty-four seven. This wasn't what I signed up for, or what Mom initially expressed she wanted, but she needed me. The variables had changed considerably. We hadn't expected a pandemic or my mother's dementia. I became my mother's helpmate, and she my dependent.

Five months earlier, September 2019, I returned to work on an alternative career path as a teacher-librarian as I completed course work and the TL certification online through Queens University. I was excited about my new job and enjoyed the work immensely. I sensed my feet were on solid ground again, and that I'd landed exactly where I was meant to be. My prayers for discernment and direction had been answered in full.

Or so I thought.

On January 27, 2020, I was placidly making dinner when a metaphorical earthquake shifted the ground beneath my feet —a 10 on the Richter scale, and beyond what I was capable of managing.

As I diced tomatoes and green onions for our Monday night meal, without warning, a telephone call would arrive from Dr. Williams, one of my neurologists. Dale had just arrived home from work, and I'd picked up Mom from her apartment. She'd been waiting in the lobby for me, as I'd pulled up to the front entry way of her apartment on my way home from my new school. This routine had been established over a year earlier. Five days a week, I picked up Mom at the Seascape Apartments where she lived independently although for how much longer was uncertain. I wondered whether I should ask

Mom to move in with us. No, not yet she wasn't ready. Nor, was I for that.

Dale and I had recently begun to reserve Wednesdays and Fridays as "date nights." After going back to work in September, I realized having Mom over for meals every night was too much. We told Mom we wanted to go out for dinner on occasion, which was true. Other nights we just needed time alone. A lie by omission seemed a good plan, in my less than assertive attempt at self-care boundaries.

Of course, Mom would tell passersby, who inquired while she sat waiting for me to pick her up, "I go to my daughters for dinner. But they don't want me on Wednesdays and Fridays."

On several occasions I'd overheard her make comments of this nature after pulling up into the fifteen-minute loading zone and exiting the car to greet her with a hug. Because of her dementia, Mom no longer realized that when I'd overhear her comment about "not being wanted," I felt wounded and defensive.

Wednesdays and Fridays, I arranged meals with printed instructions that she could warm in the microwave, up until I realized she could no longer safely operate the appliance. Without much needed resilience, I took personally what hadn't been personal.

That particular Monday night, Mom was seated in the living room watching a curling match on television while Dale sat at the kitchen table chatting with our daughter on the phone. As I stood at the chopping block whipping up a meal for my family, I free-styled and garnished a tossed salad with cranberries and slivered almonds. I assembled everything required to go with the home-cooked lasagna reheating in the oven. With the table set, I was almost ready to call everyone to the table when Apple's default ringtone interrupted an otherwise ordinary day.

~

Over the weekend, unbeknownst to me, three of my neurologists—my epileptologist, neuroimmunologist, and my movement-disorder specialist—collaborated after reading my most recent EEG. This EEG had been marked "urgent," and ordered by my epileptologist after an increased incidence of myoclonic jerks. These strange, impetuous jolts made my trunk flex backwards without warning, and had started six years earlier. Myoclonic jerks, which had started out infrequently, had now become intense and occurred much more often, resulting in a new diagnosis of orthostatic myoclonus. An even earlier EEG scan in November 2019 showed similar activity which aroused suspicion. It now seemed likely that the abnormal activity previously recorded might be the cause of the severe headaches which made it challenging to read text, concentrate while using screens, or process visual information without blinding headaches.

The most recent EEG had again recorded *abnormal* electrical activity in my prefrontal cortex, which initiated prompt actions, dialogues between specialists, and, ultimately, the phone call to unsuspecting me.

~

"As a precautionary measure, Jocelyn," my movement disorder neurologist said, as I took my phone into our bedroom for privacy, "I must advise you not to drive or work until we can complete further investigation and repeat an EEG." What I heard and internalized was: *Jocelyn, you are at considerable risk of a significant epileptic event. Your brain scan results are abnormal.* I could expect to have a seizure any day. A big one at that.

I fortified already reinforced steel walls to strengthen and defend a mind that constantly feared. It was no easy task. By muting my thoughts, could I escape further hurt? I believed the chaos happening in my body was somehow my fault, and if I didn't complain or nag about my frustration, others would accept and include me more readily. I shielded myself with silence, while inside I was filled with anger and self-pity over my new existence. Stuck, and in a fog, I was temporarily blinded to the fact that I am a child of God, loved unconditionally, and enough.

Before the twenty-seventh, I'd thought an EEG might provide updated evidence and explain what caused the exponentially increased incidence of symptoms, which prompted return visits to specialists. Changes I suspected and didn't speak of other than to practitioners. I was getting increasingly forgetful and dropping my keys too often in addition to the myoclonus. I hadn't expected or even imagined what came next.

Moments after my neurologist's call, tears leaked instinctively, while the periphery of the bedroom where I still stood blurred. I became fixated on a future robbed of self-determination.

Suddenly, I was aware for the first time that I was completely incapable of controlling my future. Impenetrable walls built to protect me from disappointment crumbled. Though I hadn't budged from where I'd taken the call, I no longer felt buttressed by a hopeful future, meaningful employment, or the freedom provided by a driver's permit. My ability to use mindfulness and create calm vanished.

Returning to the kitchen, distorted thoughts infused my pores. I began hastily devising the right words to inform Dale, without Mom learning of the significance of our conversation.

Dale was still on the phone. How he'd known to look up, while mid-sentence with Kristen that Monday night, I'm uncertain. It was uncanny. He read my face and without hesitation pulled me into his arms.

~

Dale held fast to both my hand and heart in the months ahead, although he was unaware, I journeyed down a much darker road, alone. Others sensed but didn't ask questions. Friends and colleagues weren't always in the know, or confident about what to say. So instead, they said nothing.

I believed I had everything under control. I began

tweezing my eyebrows and chin with compulsive recklessness, as I struggled to care for Mom through her cognitive decline and mourned my teaching career, which at fifty-five, I wasn't ready to let go. Simultaneously, I bore witness to my own physical, cognitive, and spiritual decline.

I held on with a death grip as my mind trash-talked. With unrealistic fears, I imagined Dale's hand loosening its grasp and his steadfast fingers no longer interlaced with mine. I asked myself repetitively, would he leave me if the medical distress became too much, or too hard? What if I could no longer meet his expectations or needs?

Might Dale vanish from our marriage, beyond the horizon like Dad, or like Mom's words and her ability to communicate? Would I be left behind, without visitors or loved ones, like so many of the elderly, who suffer distress in long-term care, alone? Would Mom feel abandoned, as I had when my father had abandoned me if I moved her to a locked-in dementia care facility?

With a forgetful mind, would she see decisions I needed to make as her power of attorney as having turned her out, or that I was no longer willing to share our home with her? I sowed seeds and catastrophized. I knew Dale had my back, but irrationally feared he might withdraw his love and leave. An ever-present possibility planted in childhood left me disbelieving of his unconditional love. I didn't trust myself or anyone else.

I had little realization of how distorted my thoughts had become in February 2020. I no longer loved who I'd become. I stopped looking at my body in the mirror; I didn't want to see her anymore. My inability to manage everything that I was trying to control impeded my ability to decide, as Mom's power of attorney, that the time had arrived to place her in long-term care. This decision came to be more than I could manage while unwell.

During this time, symbols came to represent the roller coaster of emotions I experienced. Some days, I could thrive and was a highflyer. Other days I was ashamed that I couldn't get out of bed. Every day was different. It would take a trip to Emergency at the Comox Valley Hospital, after a seven-day admission and hot-stroke-protocol, for me to realize the time to put Mom in care had passed.

Dale's hold on my heart through the spring of 2020 was a vice-grip of certainty as distorted thoughts swirled and danced with intent. Who knew "krumping" was a style of street dance? I didn't, until like a krumper, observers stared as if in a trance as I crumbled under the intense scrutiny of a mind that showed no mercy for a weary soul.

I needed help and my body was keeping score.

JOCELYN BYSTROM

# CHAPTER TWELVE

### Taps

I had a frightening dream in early June 2020.

I'd been climbing and scrambled toward a summit as I scaled an almost vertical ridge that separated two valleys. Nearing the peak there'd been fractured edges and crags which appeared insurmountable as I hunted for handholds. With intense focus, I calculated each possibility. Where might I position fingertips with certainty so as not to fall? A plummet would be deadly. I was alone in my pursuit to rise above, until I'd noticed another who climbed nearby. We each concentrated as if our lives depended on both our bravery and focus. Out of the corner of my eye I observed the other climber appeared to struggle, as I clung to maintain purchase.

My focus shifted downward once I'd found a spot to stop and rest momentarily and I noticed a woman who stood peering up at the base of the mountain. Her eyes desperately cleaved to the other climber. She held and embraced her with the sheer will of her outstretched fixation. I followed her gaze and in a fog of disbelief watched the object of her attentiveness stumble and plunge. She fell haphazardly, out of control in dream-like slow-motion, from near the dizzying height where I still clung.

The woman below ran, crossing the landscape hurriedly to reach the base of the structure, an eagle poised then swooping to catch her fallen eaglet from the nest. Then beside a mirror-like surface of pooled water, the woman stood with her arms outstretched ready to protect and cushion her beloved's fall. I hadn't thought the water's depth enough to absorb or soften the impact. Would she be killed?

I held my breath, frozen in fear, as I observed her free fall...

~

I'd stirred then awakened to another day of marking time impatiently. Suddenly alert, I didn't want to fall asleep again and re-enter the dream state. With absolute certainty I knew I didn't want to ever end up with fingers in a death grip out on a ledge. Would I have the strength to hold on? The handholds I reached for as I closed Mom's apartment of twenty-two years, grieved without support, and contemplated a life of physical decline were each difficult and more than I wanted to manage. I was losing my grip on this perilous climb. Had it simply been a dream, or rather a foreshadowing of a change of seasons?

What season was I now experiencing? Between 2014 and 2019, it had felt like one long winter, including triggering incidents, despair, darkness, and grief, with only intermittent periods of rising above and joy. Then a spring had come, a glorious season of growth and remembrance, as I looked back and reflected on my childhood and began a new therapeutic relationship with a counsellor.

But then the weather turned unpredictable. The robins had returned, but I couldn't drive anymore. The snowdrops and crocuses had bloomed, but I couldn't remember details of conversations on the telephone. I had new hope, loved my role as a teacher-librarian, and was warming up to the promise of summer. I'd been hopeful; and then I was not.

Instead of the summer I'd been longing for, another winter was on its way. A "season" which would last fourteen months between January 2020–February 2021. And to make things worse, it would occur during a worldwide pandemic. At a time when we were being bombarded with catastrophic news, a culture of fear became prevalent. I experienced social isolation and missed family and friends. Most impactfully, the possibility of testing positive for COVID-19 and death had become a worldwide reality.

My internal strength and fortitude tanked, and I constantly catastrophized. What was wrong with me? No one seemed to know. I experienced an elevated sense of urgency for answers and clarity, though the overburdened health-care system didn't seem to define 'urgency,' as I did.

I faked intelligence by compulsively recording with surgical precision every detail in a black Oxford notebook I called "My Health Journal." If asked or required to know information, I knew with certainty I would be adequately prepared with answers that made sense. This temporarily created an override of negative thoughts.

And yet, I continued to advocate for answers I believed necessary while not knowing what I needed. I pleaded, questioned, and documented instances of forgetfulness, difficult conversations, and my inability to read with ease as my eyes struggled to track from one line of text to the next. I couldn't remember anything I'd read anyway. Constant unwelcomed thoughts invaded as I worried that I, too, had dementia. I carried my notebook with a pen clipped to it, always ready.

Doctors hadn't yet determined why I was experiencing significant cognitive decline. They searched and investigated with every fibre of their beings and ordered all means of assessment.

I trusted the specialists' intention at this point as if they were gods, believing they alone were the keepers of the vault of answers I was so desperate to open. These gods I placed up on a pedestal alas were human and couldn't seem to explain the mysterious secrets of my unique body. Time after time, I'd walk away disappointed and discouraged after another appointment brought no answers.

I came to expect that any neurologist might ask me to

count backwards by sevens from two hundred with my eyes closed. This diagnostic tool first occurred in 2015 but became an incredibly difficult task for me to complete by the summer of 2020. My cognition had declined either as a side effect of medications, or my brain was simply not coding information during what appeared to be epileptic discharges specialists noted on successive EEGs.

In preparation for the backwards counting, I practiced incessantly. I knew it took ten thousand hours to master a complex skill, after reading Malcolm Gladwell's *Outliers*, so I constantly repeated this and other diagnostic tasks to not appear foolish. My health journal was ever-present with me, as I tried to memorize answers I expected would be asked.

I'd been shamed by one specialist, who hammered me with verbal mental math questions to determine if I could be distracted from the occurrence of these strange jerks, and then belittled me with cruel accusations when I didn't respond quickly or accurately. Whether I gave correct or incorrect answers, he told me I'd made errors, which confused and overwhelmed me. It didn't take long till I broke down and cried.

He'd implied as he completed his assessment that he believed I was lying about prior illicit drug use, and that there was no physical evidence for any of the symptoms I experienced.

He was pleased and smiled knowingly. I was able to stand and be distracted from experiencing myoclonic jerks.

"Really, you can't even answer basic math questions," he chided. "I thought you were a teacher who teaches math. You can't even answer simple math equations." The berating continued. "You think the correct answer to six times twelve equals seventy-two? Try again." Later, he told Dale that this was an effective way to determine whether there were underlying physical reasons rather than what he called pseudo symptoms. If I could be distracted and the jerks didn't occur while I stood unsupported, it proved that the jerks had no underlying physical cause.

I sat with shame washing over me, as he explained to my husband that this had been his intention all along. His diagnostic methods left me as raw as a freshly butchered steak.

Were the diagnostic tools by which he'd formulated his treatment plan and recommended trial of a seizure medication worth the emotional cost? They were not.

Another neurologist at a similar neurology intake used this same diagnostic with a compassionate plot twist, which enabled a surprising conflict resolution.

"Jocelyn, could you please count backwards for me inside your mind? Close your eyes, and begin at two hundred, subtracting by seven." Then she'd added, "You don't need to answer out loud, just close your eyes and complete the math in your head." I'd been incredibly relieved to do the calculations in my mind's eye although it wasn't easy. I made similar mistakes, but it didn't matter.

I did the math as asked and had been easily distracted. There was no evidence of myoclonus with this more humane approach and the results were identical. Telling diagnostic information had been successfully collected, and my shoulders released tension without tears, a sigh, or scarring. She'd earned my trust and our therapeutic relationship proceeded step by step with kindness and respect.

~

In June 2020 I prepared for an away trip to the mainland and Vancouver, for further medical assessment. My tank was empty. A three-day ambulatory EEG at Vancouver General Hospital (VGH) included daily trips to the hospital each afternoon, from where I stayed with my dear friends Rory and Cindy, to change the battery pack in the mobile recording device that recorded my brain waves. Staying with cherished friends was truly a Godsend. The EEG had been ordered by my team of neurologists to investigate further cognitive decline and increased incidence of laboured breathing. They monitored brain and body activity twenty-four seven. I hoped the investigation would provide what I desperately needed. Answers.

My neck and shoulders held stories of imagined outcomes, as I booked appointments with my massage therapist, hopeful he'd be clairvoyant, and able to read and interpret muscles stretched rigid like taffy and peanut brittle. Not knowing what eventualities, news, or outcomes I could expect from my hospital admission, I was most appreciative of a break from caregiving. I packed and prepared my backpack, doubling as an overnight bag, with extra masks, gloves, and hand sanitizer to protect against COVID-19. I took a backpack rather than a suitcase because I travelled alone at a time when only essential travel was allowed during the height of the pandemic, and prayed I'd have the strength and required peace of mind that seemed non-existent.

Were all the prerequisite details taken care of? Dale had taken time off work to stay at home and taken on caregiving responsibility for my mom, any time I needed to be absent for medical assessment. I hadn't been able to acquire necessary respite care during the pandemic; and we hadn't wanted a string of potentially virus carrying, care-partners in our home, so plans A, B, C, and D went out the window. There wasn't a line-up of caregivers willing to risk infection or responding to my desperate pleas, anyway.

Reassuring Mom, I said goodbye, hopeful she wouldn't worry. I parented an anxious child, my mother.

"Mom, I'm going to visit Kristen in Vancouver." I bent over to give her a hug as she sat viewing a pre-recorded, televised curing match. Then, to be truthful, slipping in, "I'll see my doctor while I'm there." She wouldn't understand my ill-health and medical challenges. An explanation was too complicated for an overwhelmed mind—mine, or hers.

Mom had already been robbed of vocabulary that would support meta-cognition. I constantly needed to remind her I was her daughter, Jocelyn. I'd not wanted to explain that I would be away for an undetermined number of days to travel to Vancouver for intense and invasive medical investigation. I didn't want to frighten Mom or exacerbate my own fears. Today, I'd be her care-partner, heading to Vancouver to visit her granddaughter. Perhaps, later, I'd be able to explain.

"Have a wonderful trip," Mom said, as she blew me a goodbye kiss.

Unable to drive myself to Vancouver, I'd needed an alternate plan. Dale drove me to the dedicated pickup spot in Courtenay, where Island Link picked up and transported passengers to Nanaimo, and BC Ferries' Departure Bay terminal. This bus trip would be followed by a one-and-a-half-hour ferry ride across Georgia Strait, where Rory, Cindy's spouse was scheduled to pick me up. From our home to theirs it would take five or six hours dependent on traffic and road conditions, prior to my next-day appointment to get rigged up with what I affectionately called my "brain umbilical cord" and its battery pack.

I arrived masked, gloved, and anxious about what to expect. I feared a life-threatening or shortening diagnosis, and now being exposed to the COVID-19 virus, when only essential emergency travel was allowed across British Columbia. I walked off after the ferry docked with my backpack, and in a socially distanced, single-file line of travellers, my pupils scanned constantly for the security that comes with recognition of a friendly face in a dense crowd.

This time I travelled with a cloth mask, now a mandatory requirement for essential travel, and I had chosen a heavy one, for its layered protection, however it had been incredibly difficult to breathe through. By the time I exited the terminal and walked through to the parking area I was breathing heavily and exhausted. I was grateful to recognize Rory, standing by his parked car, waving his arms to draw my attention. His welcoming smile was a bright light.

Each time I'd needed to travel for medical investigation between January and June to see various specialists my travel had fallen into a similar, repetitive pattern. Reaching their home, I'd head to bed for a nap, happily ensconced in what had come to be affectionately known as *"my room,"* in my home away from home. After napping, I stayed up way too late enjoying the freedom and respite of what felt like a mini vacation.

Later, far past my usual 10 p.m. bedtime, I'd fall exhausted into bed after adding distilled water to my continuous positive airway pressure (CPAP) machine tank and don the nasal mask I'd used since it was recommended to improve the quality of my sleep. Then despite the lateness of the hour, I lay awake with an anxious busy brain too supercharged to sleep.

My epileptologist had referred me earlier to a neuro-sleep specialist, and I'd begun using a CPAP machine, usually used for obstructive apnea. In my case, I surmised, she'd hoped the machine would help regulate my sleep and reduce the frequency of severe migraine-like headaches. Dale and I both now used CPAP machines, side by side at night, while we slept. I'd desperately hoped her suggestion would work.

I was grateful to be dropped off at the hospital's front doors the following day by Cindy. I entered the hospital alone since family members weren't allowed to accompany patients during Stage One pandemic protocols. This was another reason Dale hadn't accompanied me. Safety measures were being strictly enforced at the front entrance, as I'd entered for the initial six-hour-long EEG and set up for the three-day ambulatory EEG. Later, I'd text Cindy for a ride back to their place. After the third and final day of monitoring I decided to stay an extra night after Cindy offered to drive me to the ferry for the return trip home to Comox the following morning rather than immediately after picking up as was originally planned.

I wasn't ready to return and magical thinking made it seem a holiday. Strings of guilt rather than pearls encircled my neck.

The next day, back home in Comox, I entered through

doors I'd chosen when we'd renovated our house. I climbed the interior stairs of our split-level home and then turned at the top. Mom, still seated in her favourite recliner, was watching another curling match.

"Hello Mom, I'm home from Vancouver."

She still recognized me, and responded, "How was your trip? Did you have a wonderful time?"

"I enjoyed a visit with Kristen, yet I'm happy to be home." Is compassionate deception still lying? To whom was the compassion addressed or required? To whom was I sparring unnecessary distress?

~

A couple days later, my epileptologist called to report that the most recent EEG showed no changes, and that "abnormal discharges" were still occurring. They were still seeing epileptiform-appearing spikes and discharges between one-half to eight seconds in length seconds in length. No answers yet. *Did I have epilepsy or not?*

By July 2020, most days I simply sat, reclined, or slept.

~

The investigative journey continued. A neuroimmunologist ordered a lumbar puncture, also known as a spinal tap, to be completed July 20 in Vancouver at the University of British Columbia's Parkinson's Clinic by yet another neurologist who my neuroimmunologist reassured me was highly skilled. After arranging the appointment, he told me, "In all honesty, it can be painful."

He wasn't wrong.

I prepared myself as I usually had with positivity and prayer. I believed, after reading online that spinal taps were often completed to diagnose serious and life-threatening conditions after researching what to expect during the procedure. I learned that a hollow needle would be inserted into the space surrounding the spinal column in my lower back to withdraw cerebrospinal fluid (CSF), and that CSF is a clear fluid that bathes and cushions the brain and spinal cord. Spinal fluid is produced by the body continuously and then reabsorbed by the brain. Spinal fluid cells, which include water, proteins and sugars are essential to maintain balance in the nervous system.

It was obvious to me that something was extremely out of whack with my nervous system. I was terrified of the lumbar puncture procedure, of what they'd find, and what it might mean.

I first became petrified of needles as a kid, after falling off my reconditioned, but new to me, banana bike. A bicycle Mom gifted to me for my ninth birthday. When the spring weather had finally been good enough to try it out, I'd followed Sandra, my big sister, as we peddled down the steep, curvy hill on our way to play at Puntledge Park.

My new bike was pink with a sparkly seat and shiny pink streamers that I loved. It had tall handlebars that were hard for me to reach, an elongated seat and a sissy bar. The wheel at the front was super small, tiny compared to the fatter, larger tire on the back. I didn't really like riding the bike because it was hard to pedal and steer, but I hadn't wanted to tell Mom. I knew it was probably expensive. I did love those pink streamers with the silvery glitter on three different tints of pink.

I'd been peddling to catch up while racing downhill, when I swerved to avoid a small stone. Next, the handlebars were ripped from my small hands, and I flew over the bike. I blacked out. The next thing I remember was my face and hands leaking blood into someone's sink and the water coloured darker than my streamers.

Afterwards, the doctor who looked at my scrapes and scratches strongly recommended that Mom bring me back to the hospital's lab in a few days. He mentioned something about a "blood test" and "checking for infection."

"They'd draw blood . . . there'd be a needle," Mom said, as we got into the car headed to the hospital. *They're going to take my blood out?* How would they do that? The doctor had recommended that both my sister and me have a blood test.

"She could have passed on the infection," he'd said. How I'd wondered? Her blood was going to be in me. I couldn't believe it. I hadn't known then that bacteria was so hardy, lives on the skin naturally, or that it can enter the bloodstream through a wound causing sepsis.

When we returned to the hospital Friday after mom got off work, the lab tech thought herself very clever. She suggested Sandra go first. I'd been reluctant and hadn't cooperated when the nurse called my name, afraid of getting the needle Mom had explained we'd be getting. Still, I wasn't convinced that Sandra, if she went first, would say it hurt. She doesn't always tell me everything.

Mom went in with Sandra while I waited on the bench just outside the door with Mom's purse. I decided not to stick around to find out if it would be less painful than I imagined.

I'm that little girl, you know the naughty one with the curl, in Longfellow's poem that Mom used to read from the book of nursery rhymes:

> There was a little girl,
> And she had a little curl
> Right in the middle of her forehead.
> When she was good
> She was very, very good,
> And when she was bad, she was horrid.

I took the car keys from Mom's purse, ran to the car, and locked myself in. By the time my sister and Mom came outside to find me it had been too late to resume the appointment and my mom too embarrassed by my behaviour to return inside. I was proud of myself and didn't mind that only my sister got to pick out a special prize at the store for being so brave.

~

Still not a fan of needles in 2020, I'd Googled what to expect when having a lumbar puncture.

The research, while informative, seemed grim and hadn't adequately prepared me for the reality of what was to come.

~

It's difficult to write about pain, terror, and losing control. I avoided reliving the incident and initially hadn't wanted to record it in writing. Looking back, I realize that I nearly lost my mind on that table during the procedure and was grateful that despite COVID protocols Kristen was allowed to accompany and be present with me during the procedure.

I mentally escaped, faster than the hammer action of a sprinter's legs, kicking out from the starting blocks. With my eyes glazed over I took off to where I had a bird's eye view of myself, and to a place more remote than my conscious mind or abilities could fathom.

My mind sought a place free of unexpected outcomes as physical pain inflicted horror like I'd never experienced previously. I travelled, remote from my body to a place from where in my mind's eye I could look down from in safety and observe. Seeing, where I lay in a fetal position, tightly wrapped, cocooned by my own arms and no others. I sensed my daughter's eyes as she watched and witnessed my terror.

What was she seeing? The first, second, third, and fourth lumbar punctures had been unsuccessful, and they attempted a fifth. From above I wondered if she saw what I did? Her mother no longer inhabiting her body, frozen in time and space and incapable of prayer. Did she know that hope was a non-existent ally and had vanished, as she watched me as I lay tense and rigid. Did she hear fear reign as the crowned champion as I instinctually assumed the fetal position with my back curved forward, legs brought up tightly against my abdomen, head bowed, and eyes forced shut.

Looking back, I see an instinctual reaction to the extreme stress my brain was no longer capable of coping with, a soul in shreds. My daughter later told me, "I threw up, then swallowed the vomit back down, as I watched."

Remembering now, I'm back on that metallic silver table, dressed only in a hospital gown and my underwear. Jockey's, lowered to create the requested room, a sterile place, along my spine. My skin now reddened by preparation and process. They've assured a sterile puncture zone, up and down my spinal cord. Knots in the gown, hung untied. Others were tied tightly within. These existed and doubled, as tension gathered each sinew into fists of exertion.

The fifth attempt was also unsuccessful, as they hit bone.

"Let's try another day with fluoroscopy," someone said as multiple voices filled the space. *Fluoroscopy*? Internal knots persisted. Tightened screws inscribed fear and stripped me bare.

Then someone was saying: "You can get dressed and go now." Immobilized I wondered how I could possible compose myself or get dressed? Numb, I heard, "You're good to go."

Curled there, I whimpered, "I need a minute."

"Take your time" were their last words as doctors left the room.

My daughter and I were left alone in their wake, I'd been speechless yet grateful to not be alone. Kristen came to me immediately—caressing, calming, gathering, and nurturing. She cared. Our roles, reversed. She'd become the parent. And I, the child.

Months later, she reminded me, "This is our thing, Mom. When I was young, you came to all my appointments at Children's Hospital, and now, I come to yours." I couldn't believe, it. What had I done to deserve such a generous-hearted child? How was it possible that this beautiful, intelligent, capable, wise daughter was mine?

God uniquely knit her together, His beloved, in my womb.

Not even a month later, more frightening symptoms would emerge.

JOCELYN BYSTROM

# CHAPTER THIRTEEN

**The Cost of Caring**

In the confines of our homes, the pandemic put daily life as we knew it on hold. Lockdowns became a new reality as fear mounted and we watched the worldwide death toll climb exponentially. I awakened in early July 2020 to another unprecedented winter. It would be a season measured by love, sadness, anger and feeling overwhelmed. As the world began to reconnect through Zoom and other online platforms, my neurologist referred me to the University of British Columbia's brain health and wellness programming. Classes were available on Zoom. Through the UBC Brain Wellness Program I found support I hadn't known I desperately needed.

Mentors and instructors diligently rebuilt circuitry for willing participants with brain health challenges. Together, we learned tools for building resilience. I can't say enough about the implicit value these programs had when I was at an all-time spiritual low. I hadn't realized how emphatically my body and mind sought nourishment and inspiration.

I took a leap of faith and signed up for an art therapy class titled "Art with Heart." I registered based solely on a small increment of trust my movement disorder neurologist had earned. In addition, I signed up for a writing class. I clung to the fact that no previous writing experience was necessary, and that the class was specifically aimed to support individuals who struggled with chronic brain health. I hadn't imagined it possible that through art I would discover a miniscule spark. Or that through online classes my body might be able to express itself through an exploration of colour and with the guidance of a mindful and collaborative therapist.

Was it possible that if I fanned the tiny flame my body and mind would dare to hope?

Each "Art with Heart" therapy session began with an exploratory prompt or check-in. My first art therapy class was to create a personalized mandala. The following week we listened to a guided exploration over Zoom, which anchored and grounded us. While we attended to our breathing, we were asked to consider gratitude and bring something or someone to mind.

My daughter Kristen came to mind instantly. It had only been a few days since the traumatic lumbar puncture experience, when she had literally and prayerfully been there for me. I listened to the instructor with conscious intention and a strong desire for healing. I also sought my inner voice, which we were told would most likely have something to say to us about gratitude, as we began the process of artmaking.

I instinctively drew curvy, overlapping lines with a thick black Sharpie, then added layers of red to shapes that emerged. Blood red to represent pain, fear, and my body's distress. I coloured in sections of the page symbolizing where Kristen and I had been seated. Where Kristen had been I added joyful colours of gratitude: yellow, orange, pink, and sky blue. Then I surrounded these with red for the pain I believed I caused her as she witnessed mine. The continuous, spiral-like waves threaded around two side-by-side pages in my sketchbook. Many of these appeared as teardrop shaped and these I filled with light blue—a colour which brought light, lift, and calm, and was guided by my intuition. Was this to be a work of art that enabled me to discharge the frozen fear and energy my body still held?

As I told the therapist what the art process recalled, we

discussed the art through a lens of distance. I was able to discharge and release at least a little of the dread that lingered.

~

Although it seemed like no one was noticing, that wasn't true. Dale noticed. But perhaps he didn't know how to articulate the mental health concerns he witnessed or hadn't wanted to layer additional worry on top of the physical chaos. My children were attentive as well.

Yet I'd needed the *doctors* to take notice. By not being alert, or tuned into the fact that my fear was compounding, no one was adapting to what was happening.

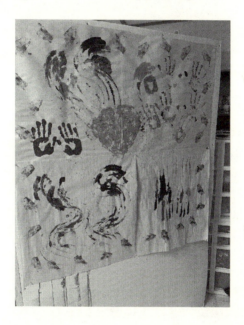

One of my therapeutic artistic creations after a day filled with seizures. I let my body speak up and choose its colors and expressions.

I needed medical practitioners who noticed and adapted their diagnostic processes to include mental health assessment. I required doctors, specialists, therapists, and practitioners to observe, listen, and note rather than continue to refer me for specialized physical examination and assessment. Perhaps they might have given audience to what the body was saying. No one advocated for mental health support during the initial phases of diagnostic assessment until late July 2020.

At times, I could stand back and explore what my art was telling me. All that was required of me in art therapy classes was that I pay attention to my feelings and match what I found in colour and form. However, I often got sidetracked as I experienced physical, cognitive, and spiritual decline, which I continued to compulsively record.

~

Catastrophic thoughts continued to spiral out of control as I learned to express angst with paint and use guided writing under the tutelage of skilled instructors. One facilitated my learning of the Intensive Journaling process, first trademarked by Ira Progoff, to provide release for minds heavily taxed by traumatic incidents. I slowly gave myself permission to feel and worked diligently to tune into my body's needs. For the first time in months I recognized new sparks of hope.

After I witnessed those initial catalysts, I deduced that I had nothing to lose by fanning the flame. My pen floated freely across the page, as I unleashed words to bear witness to what my body needed to express. The writing, like those first paintings, was chaotic and messy. Like when I'd scraped hands and fingernails through black and red paint and dredged paint across the page, making the sound of nails on the chalkboard. It wasn't pretty. I threw and spattered colour recklessly, freed of all confines. I let go of judgement of the product and created as I learned this art was about the process. Art therapy while I was in crisis was a Godsend.

Mentors and instructors created brave spaces for uncertain overwhelmed minds. Ever so gently I caressed trust and allowed myself to feel. I acknowledged that it was okay to not be okay, and acceptable to express rage, uncertainty, and sadness. It took time, courage, vulnerability, and letting go of beliefs which no longer served wellness to fan the sparks. I couldn't trust easily during those summer months of uncertainty.

As I moved through this bleak season of prolonged waiting for diagnostic clarity and caregiving for my mother in our home, I was angled toward illness and struggled with my mental health. All I saw was my physical deterioration and the uncertainty of knowing my future would no longer be what I'd hoped and dreamed through the years. I was unaware of my monocular vision as I gazed unknowingly through a kaleidoscope void of colour.

Meanwhile, my tormented mind wandered and lost its way.

~

What did my mom think about when she'd been fifty-six? Did she worry about what lay ahead or was in the rear view mirror? Was her mind spinning and spiraling like mine? Were her shoulders overburdened by distorted thoughts?

Mom, what questions caused your catastrophic thoughts and fortune-telling when at forty-seven and a single mother, you waited up at night for me to come home from a date? I judged you harshly for what I believed was needless anxiety. At seventeen, I was surprised and confused when you asked me, "Did he hurt you?" as I stepped through our front door after an exhilarating Friday night at the drive-in theatre's double feature with my first boyfriend.

Was that *your* experience while dating, Mom? Why couldn't you have simply asked, "Did you have a good time, Jocelyn?" And then welcomed me home with affection. The following summer, in 1982, I began dating Dale. At eighteen, I continued to stare into Mom's fearful eyes, unable to comprehend that the body keeps score.

~

In 2020, I peered into Mom's vacant eyes and witnessed a mouth and mind robbed of words and language. I began to comprehend the cruelty of her having had no one to bear witness to her longings or sorrows. I was able to acknowledge that my life differed dramatically from my mother's. I had the stability of Dale: life partner and husband. He'd chosen me, committed daily to express his love, and walked alongside me. His actions generated a more secure lens of safety and *us*, while my body continued to experience physical and emotional decline.

Choosing a lens of gratitude enabled me to begin to navigate the trauma my body held. With a lens of appreciation for the support I had and limited spiritual belief I clung to, it had been enough. I was unconditionally loved by God, worthy and enough.

Dale showered me with acts of service and generosity, and I sensed love through these expressions. His actions held my unglued mind secure, while God held me in my brokenness, and loved me anyway. Even when I was incapable of using Dale's love language to gift him love in return, he held me close.

I wanted to live.

Fortunately, it was not my experience to consider or attempt suicide. I did, however, catastrophize about my death. I imagined it in gruesome horrific detail, and routinely awoke from terrifying nightmares of being pursued. Though unaware in July, I was held by my loving Heavenly Father, unlike the earthly one who had abandoned me. God held my heart and loved me unconditionally. I wasn't worthy but loved regardless. All I needed to do was believe I was His Beloved child. I did, and I do. Even when I walked in discouragement and darkness, unable to see a spark of hope, God held his beloved secure and guarded my heart and mind.

~

As August approached, medications continued to make me cognitively fuzzy. Unlike the confident, capable, intelligent women I believed I used to be. I was ashamed when I looked at the girl in the mirror. I asserted myself with neurologists and teams of experts when I required them to rethink unsuccessful medication trials, but not for the girl in the mirror. That girl's voice had been silenced.

When I looked in the mirror, I saw someone I didn't recognize, and with condescension asked, *What have you let happen to yourself?* She didn't answer. Instead, she'd look sullenly back at me with judgement.

The girl in the mirror grew wearier by the day, her eyes hollow with fear and trepidation about what to expect next. The stress of unexplained body sensations, migraine headaches, and chronic back pain were the result of endless myoclonic jerks as she waited months between appointments. That girl, the girl in the mirror, was overindulging. She'd eaten seconds of homemade macaroni and cheese, extra slices of freshly baked bread slathered in butter, and double scoops of chocolate chip ice cream. All these now hopelessly hung on her hips and thighs.

I wasn't even hungry. Her hazel eyes cried out with regret. Ashamed.

I wandered sluggishly from the bathroom and discovered more uncertainty each day. I'd forgotten routines and was without an authentic purpose. I put on over thirty pounds. I couldn't bear to whisper "two hundred" out loud ... then "two hundred and two." I judged myself harshly and believed others observed, judged, and cringed not knowing how to encourage or respond. As I struggled during the pandemic, with layer upon layer of traumatic loss and without emotional resilience, those around me were traumatized by the physical manifestations of my struggle with mental health and illness.

I became unable to participate in conversations due to an inability to hear or code what I'd heard. I experienced short intervals of hearing deficiency and alarming changes in my cognitive ability, which left me unable to remember details, or hold information on the tabletop of my memory. Questions asked, I missed. What I'd wanted to express was forgotten. When an appropriate lull in conversation created an opportunity for connection or a polite opening to speak, I couldn't remember vital details. I now feared a diagnosis of dementia more than anything.

Cognitive loss robbed me of confidence, drive, passion, and joy. Intuitive friends and family witnessed shocking changes that didn't require a specialist to observe. They saw, heard, and experienced their loved one's personality, mind, secure faith, and inability to move efficiently, and grew silent with concern. At the rate of my decline, some even wondered if I would live to see 2021. All the while I was aware of the strain I caused and carried additional guilt.

I needed someone to respectfully say, "I see you're struggling, Jocelyn, and can't imagine what you're going through." Followed by, "But I want you to know I care. Can you tell me about your struggles?"

I needed to explain that in the doctor's office I'd been ashamed after reading the BMI (body mass index) chart, before shamefully looking away. Embarrassed, like when I pretended years earlier to be looking at whatever else was beside the period pads or tampons at the drug store. Someone might see me buy an "unmentionable," as my mother spoke of them, and judge me, as she had when she once found tampons in the bathroom cupboard which she hadn't purchased. "You aren't using *those*, are you?" she asked.

The options didn't seem great when the only choices had been sanitary pads that leaked or having nothing at all. I hadn't been taught about menstruation or known to be prepared or expect to need period supplies. I arrived home too often needing something "unmentionable" and found nothing helpful under the bathroom sink. We didn't talk about unmentionable things.

The chart in the doctor's office informed me I was morbidly obese. I was ashamed that the suggested goal weight for my height apparently was impossible for me to achieve. I knew this... having tried so very many times to lose weight unsuccessfully without support or appropriate knowledge.

Obesity would be just one more label I acquired without effort and couldn't control. Until I did, and then I controlled my food intake like a religious zealot. I'd successfully achieve my goal weight, only to gain it back slowly, beginning a vicious cycle I repeated endlessly ever since moving out and living alone at seventeen to attend university. It was apparent that I required a lifelong commitment to scamper endlessly on the dieting hamster wheel.

Again, I needed someone to notice, to observe my struggle and ask repeatedly what my experiences of living were like. Until I learned to trust, I needed others to listen with curiosity and compassion. Someone? Anyone. Who would be willing to take the time, learn mental health first aid, and initiate a supportive conversation?

I needed to believe they cared, would listen without judgement, and hear without trying to fix what I believed was unfixable. I needed to believe I had value, was loved and worthy of their time. It takes time to listen with your heart, to be fully present for someone and to sit in the discomfort of what's uncomfortable. It takes compassion to listen without robbing you of your grief, or to maintain and uphold the belief that you're capable and strong enough to swim in grief's waves and find your way back to the shore in your own time.

I longed to be heard, believed, and worthy of care. Care I didn't lavish on myself or believe myself important enough to prioritize.

A voice in my head constantly reminded me, *I want her back—the Jocelyn from before the tightly knotted weave of traumatic incidents.*

I heard myself advocate for her as I reached, grasped for, and articulated my needs to specialists. I heard myself explain repetitively that my body wasn't managing, that the taste of fear made low-calorie sodas seem toxic with a chemical taste in my mouth. The longer my smell and taste stimuli were impeded by stress, the more diminished my ability to find food pleasing became.

It didn't stop my body from sending the *I'm hungry* signal though . . . as I ate and ate and ate.

I believed erroneously that I could control my fear and tears. I wouldn't let others see and escaped to a safe, private space to dissolve into a puddle. *Don't let anyone find out that you're weak, vulnerable, and an imposter*, continued to be my mantra. I wasn't capable, hadn't managed for a long time, but was an expert at flying under the radar. Or so I thought. To date, no one had found out that I wasn't highly skilled or the most capable person in the room to teach or complete what was expected of me as an educational professional.

Then I'd made the fatal error.

I'd shown my vulnerability, and in weakness and a state of shock written a letter and pressed send.

The only thing I seemed to remember was that they'd found out my truth. I was an imposter. I'd been discovered, judged, and found wanting. Nothing else mattered and no one seemed to care or understand the gravity of the loss or grief I lived with.

My motto became more deeply etched: *Control, hide, protect, and shelter your heart at any cost.*

The toll of caring exacted an exorbitant cost. I believed I was weak, disabled, and that my emotional battery would always be empty. I apparently wasn't worthy of the time, energy, or words of affirmation I longed for to discharge the big feelings and scary emotions instinctively arising from my reptilian brain. I was unable to refill my mental health reservoir. It became difficult to believe I could trust others or that anyone wanted to take the time or cared. Distorted thoughts prevailed. Perceived stigma, like the knowledge that a virus could infiltrate a compromised immune system, exacerbated my inability to trust.

Control became my friend, knowing I could trust myself to guard my heart when unconditional love was bound to be withdrawn. I'd been found lacking. I had an encapsulated fear of bad events which I believed would happen unless I took preventative action.

Pre-emptively, I'd control the narrative and defend pre-existing wounds whose scar tissue dulled my confidence and instilled armour. Not trusting or expressing emotion became an unwritten, unacknowledged childhood strategy early and had served me well then. But it no longer served healthy communication on which adult relationships grow, thrive, and are restored.

No one asked: *What's that like for you?*

Another specialist called. I'd waited for the call after being referred in June for a mammogram. "We need to rule out cancer." Dale saw the emotional cost as I heard these words and was now masterful at interpreting my body language. He'd known this would be yet another tipping point. There were too many in short order to process or survive. He interpreted my emotional anguish though I couldn't manage to talk about it. Dale witnessed eyes glazing over, taut shoulders, and an increased frequency of loud sighs.

He listened, noticed, and without reservation shouldered the mantle of care-partner for both my mother and me, all whilst I still erroneously believed I was my mom's capable caregiver. Each time my neurologist called, Dale at my side was an invested, supportive care-partner.

Imagine bracing your already compromised mind and body for the possibility of battling cancer? Dale proofread emails as I experienced complete and utter certainty and proof that I was no longer capable to proofread and double-check my writing for typos, grammatical errors, or to discern whether what I'd written even made sense. Emails detailed elevated fear, the increased tension held in my body and frightening sensations which fully electrified my circuitry. My body had become intensely emotionally charged, without a relief valve, and my health diary overflowed with page after page of details I no longer trusted my brain to remember.

My mind simply couldn't comprehend what my body

knew. Where might we find a fortune teller to answer questions burned into my psyche about my body's hidden secrets? Who if anyone could solve this expert level Mensa puzzle and release me from Pandora's box?

Escape, I believed, was no longer a viable option as I became a prisoner of my brain's cleverly mixed up, erroneous messages.

And then my body took charge, signalling it would not be denied. In the early morning of July 25, I experienced a thunderclap headache during intimacy which felt like a ruptured blood vessel in my brain above my left eye.

It was a ten out of ten on the pain scale—intense, brief, and terrifying.

It dissipated rapidly, so I was able to convince Dale I didn't require a trip to the hospital. Embarrassment was capable of closeting away rationality and common sense, and I feared discussions about sexual intimacy and my perceived sexual inadequacy. Intimacy took a back seat to fear. I became increasingly uncertain about when I could expect seizures during sex.

Why did discussing intimacy feel strictly taboo? Was my fear a holdover from early thoughts of sex as unmentionable. Did my reptilian brain fear abandonment if I discussed what I believed was strictly private? What happened in my prefrontal cortex as I became frozen with fear and each seizure began? Words evaporated. Thoughts raced. It was inextricably difficult to imagine a resolution to any conversation which didn't end with Dale leaving me. I believed with complete certainty that when a man's needs aren't met, they'd seek to have those needs met elsewhere—with someone else. Catastrophic thoughts drained me of assertiveness and big-picture thinking. My anxious brain couldn't provide a rational explanation that proved Dale wouldn't leave me.

After lunch that same day my thoughts were caught in a *What if?* gridlock.

While Keith, Kristen and Mom sat in the living room I

headed to my writing room, which used to be my sewing room and a place of creativity and joy. I used to quilt; sew handbags, wallets, and purses; play with fabric, and create gifts others delighted in receiving. In 2020, the space was solely a place to find solace, one of very few rooms that were not shared common spaces. It was a place to shelter where I could be alone with my thoughts. Seated at my sewing table, then doubling as a writing table, I experienced a massive tingling sensation in my face. After the unforeseen terrifying headache this morning I believed it was time to tell Dale I might in fact need to get checked out.

I headed to the kitchen and whispered in Dale's ear, "Come with me," as I gestured with my pointer finger for him to follow me. He made a joke about hoping we were heading to the bedroom, but I led him back into my sewing room across the hall from the room typically reserved for the three S's: sleep, sex, and sickness. Dale followed me into the tight space I'd sequestered as mine and asked, "What's up?"

After I explained that I was again experiencing tingling in my face and now also my fingers, he made the decision.

"It's time. I'm taking you to Emergency." Dale's a take-control kind of guy in a chaotic situation, and all hell was breaking loose. It's what he does masterfully well as a businessman.

I went in search of my cell phone and coat as Dale left to talk to the kids. Kristen was then twenty-three, and Keith twenty-six, but they would always be our "kids" in my mind. We agreed to meet back at the front door ASAP.

When ready I went to join Dale and was surprised to overhear him saying, "Mom and I are going to run some errands. We'll be back in a bit."

With that we headed out to the car and off to the Comox Valley's hospital ER. On the way, I experienced extreme fatigue, shortness of breath, and the tingling escalated. I wouldn't realize till later that I was experiencing a panic attack.

Instead, as I exited the car at Emergency during pandemic protocols, Dale was told not to get out of the car and that I was to walk to a waiting wheelchair. When I couldn't walk and struggled to exit the car, Dale got out anyway and supported me as I walked with considerable effort and finally dropped into the waiting chair. After an extremely quick assessment, I heard, "Code ___" (I don't remember the colour), followed by "Hot-Stroke Protocol required." And then everything got exponentially intense.

A wave of chaos surrounded me and triggered additional trauma as highly skilled, trained experts proactively trained to save lives, took over.

# CHAPTER FOURTEEN

### Aftermath and Admission

Late on the twenty-fifth, the internal medicine specialist in communication with a neurologist in Victoria communicated their belief that I had experienced a minor stroke. I was admitted to the second-floor surgical recovery unit since our local hospital didn't have a neurology department. Through the night, I was awakened regularly for neurological assessments.

"What's this?" I was asked. "And this?" as I identified picture after picture.

"What month is it? And year?" I was asked to describe what was wrong with the cookie jar picture. Then asked to read a short passage. Both of which I could do. Then came the pinpoint flashlight in the eyes as they assessed visual fields and pupillary light reflex. Next came the ability to follow the "H" pattern and facial sensation tests using a sharp object to lightly prick the face, torso, and limbs. This would help specialists I later learned to determine whether my challenges were in the cerebral cortex, thalamus, or sensory pathways of the brain, spinal cord, or peripheral nerves.

With each poke I was asked: "Sharp or dull?"

My hearing was assessed, followed by an assessment of tone in all four limbs for strength. "Say *ahhh*." Then the reflex hammer came out to test deep tendon reflexes.

Finally, the neurological assessments would end after

the finger to nose test when I was expected to extend my arm and touch the neurologist's finger and then my nose repeatedly as they moved their finger to different locations.

*Phew.* I seemed to have passed. I attempted sleep while listening to ringing, beeping, and screeching alarms as my roommates were assessed post-surgery. Fifty-nine minutes later, they'd return with the cookie jar picture, and this routine played out repeatedly that first night with slight variations.

By morning, one of my roommates was to be discharged, another had been admitted during the night, and flashing lights besides alarms continued to beep on various monitors, mine and theirs. Just after four in the morning, an ER nurse showed up to remove my Holter monitor, a portable electrocardiogram (ECG) used to record my heart's electrical activity continuously for the first twenty-four hours. The portable ECG monitor, I overheard, was needed in the emergency department; and shouldn't have come with me to the surgical unit, the ER nurse explained to the surgical unit attendant.

My busy brain took in all kinds of extraneous details as I listened rather than slumbered. I had heard no answers or even clues that I'd needed or listened for. What was wrong with me? Why had I experienced a minor stroke? I'd been told to expect the possibility of a significant neurological event ... but thought they meant a seizure. When would I be discharged? Could Dale bring me things I needed, like toiletries and warm socks? My feet and toes were cold as ice, and I required ear plugs. I truly needed to dull the constant bombardment of sound to get some sleep.

Fortunately, Dale had forgotten his iPad in the ER, which helped me pass the sleepless hours until the battery died. I hoped my phone, which by six in the morning was letting me know it, too, needed to be charged would hold out as I waited to call Dale at a time I knew he would be up. Our alarm goes off daily at 5:45 a.m. though we rarely get up promptly.

Unbeknownst to me, Dale had already anticipated and

delivered a large emergency kit. Before 8 a.m., two very large and heavy bags with my first and last name printed on 8 x 11" printer paper were delivered, containing everything I'd hoped for and more. Tucked in with the necessities were additional creature comforts, including chocolate sweets, a bottle of Mrs. Dash to supplement otherwise bland hospital food, and my personal favourite, red, strawberry licorice.

A handmade card Kristen tucked in made me cry. As I read the just right words she'd selected to encourage and reassure, tears of gratitude flowed. Their care package made all the difference.

I was no longer alone with my catastrophic thoughts in a hospital room full of unanswered questions. I could connect, communicate, and despite pandemic protocols, draw close to my family. Now that I had what I deemed the necessities: chargers, a toothbrush and toothpaste, wool socks and cozy slippers, art supplies and my sketchbook—in addition to my laptop—I experienced a growing sense of confidence that I would manage and arrive home to loving arms.

My compassionate, generous-hearted best friend who'd asked me out on that first date, river tubing on the Pembina River, still had my back. And he remembered to pack my favourite fleece pajamas.

It was painful to have the adhesive patches which secured the ECG electrodes removed. Five red patches of inflamed skin remained after they were withdrawn from my torso and limbs. It seemed that I was that one-in-a-million patient who experienced the dreaded adverse reactions television commercials report in fine print. I was that person who'd get all those scary side effects. Medications that 99 percent of the population benefitted from, my body didn't appreciate. Just my luck!

Day after day, the internal medicine specialist overseeing my care arrived mid-morning to repeat a neurological exam, ask questions and debrief what had been learned. She'd told me to expect my admission post-stroke would be at least a week.

"Not much will happen over the weekend," she'd said. I'd been admitted to ER on a Friday night and the "emergency" was over. Now the waiting had begun.

With too much time and not enough to do, my busy brain manically conjectured in a state of hyper-arousal. Visitors weren't allowed under any circumstances this early in 2020. Pandemic protocols ensured I was safe from the dreaded virus, but not distorted thoughts.

On Monday, July 27, I had one assessment after another, which included drop-ins from a social worker who'd asked about my caregiving responsibilities for Mom, and medical residents who were curious to listen and learn about this unprecedented, strange individual and event which was now being questioned. And later in the day, by a physiotherapist and an occupational health practitioner. *Had it been a stroke or not?*

Initially, I tried to keep track of all these assessments in my health journal, which Dale had sent in the care package. I couldn't keep track of it all and gave up trying. Perhaps I needed to trust the doctors and nurses for my care, at least a little.

It was decided collaboratively among specialists that I would have the repeat lumbar puncture they'd spoken of in June. "Might as well," the internal medicine specialist suggested. "You're going to be in hospital hanging out waiting for other assessments, anyway."

I understood the logic, but this didn't mean I wasn't terrified after the previously failed attempts to collect a sample of lumbar fluid and rule out if I had an autoimmune disorder. My neuroimmunologist from UBC wanted to determine If I had any unique antibodies warring with my immune system. Was that what was causing autoimmune encephalitis and/or an unexpected cancer involving my brain and spinal cord?

The only good news—the second attempt at the lumbar

puncture would be "with fluoroscopy."

"Can you please explain how that works?" I asked. "How is 'with fluoroscopy' different from without?" *I knew what without was like!*

It was explained that a fluoroscopy-guided lumbar puncture used an imaging tool that enabled the radiologist to look at moving body structures, like an X-ray movie. A contrast dye would help the radiologist see my spine-surrounding nerves as he inserted the hollow needle in my lower back to withdraw cerebrospinal fluid.

That answered my question, but hardly relieved my fears.

My priest called while I was waiting to be transported to the surgical unit for this latest lumbar procedure.

"Is it okay to be calling you now, Jocelyn?" she asked. "A friend of yours called to let me know you'd been admitted to the ER." I was surprised to be getting this call from our priest. I hadn't yet spoken face to face with our new priest, who'd only recently been recruited from Wales to replace our previous pastor, who was on medical leave.

She asked a few additional questions to break the ice before it occurred to me—I had a decision to make. Would I trust and tell her the truth or respond with my usual quip, "I'm fine?"

I realized it was time to be honest and express my fears. If not to a priest, then to whom? No one previously had explicitly asked.

I'd needed someone to ask but hadn't trusted anyone yet with the answers.

What's it been like, since you lost your treasured career in gifted education, experienced debilitating physical symptoms and cognitive decline, and were finally told you could no longer work?

Wasn't anyone curious to know how it felt to have experienced this magnitude of stress and been told repetitively that my EEG reports showed abnormal findings? Perhaps they might have inquired, saying, "I can't imagine, what's it like for you to be a full-time care-partner to your mother with dementia; and also, be unable to work or drive?"

*Could they even imagine the dark place I now dwelled?* Was I simply having a self-pity party? Did I need to build a bridge and suck it up? Their silence, I imagined, spoke volumes, and told me friends were too busy. I perceived that checking in with a toxic friend like me had become a noxious experience. Distorted thoughts clouded my judgement, and side effects of medication further impaired my discernment.

Is this what it's like when death comes calling during a pandemic? The priest calls, heart and Bible in hand, praying and providing last rights at your bedside. *How ill am I?*

After her call, I'd been grateful for a measure of peace while she prayed for me over the phone. I looked forward to meeting her in person someday. Maybe? It felt wonderful to have had someone who'd listened and expected nothing in return. She hadn't been fearful of sitting in discomfort with me while I finally voiced my fears and concerns. I emitted a loud sigh of relief sensing that those fears I'd voiced aloud had escaped my mind.

But the measure of peace didn't last as I was wheeled to radiology shortly thereafter. Fear reigned supreme.

The repeat lumbar puncture, with fluoroscopy, short hours after the priest's call was an entirely unique experience. It couldn't have differed more rigorously from the invasive outpatient procedure the month prior. For that I was sincerely grateful.

The second attempt was more than a successful procedure. The radiologist collected the required spinal fluid, which enabled blood technicians the clarity of a negative result. Specialists communicated that they'd been able to rule out both epilepsy and cancer.

*Hallelujah!*

Next in line was a repeat ECG. Afterwards, I sketched

with felt pens lovingly packed by Dale. I was inspired to document this opposite experience of undergoing a lumbar puncture and wished to visually record my experience in hope of capturing the fleeting phenomena and multisensory response this latest procedure had evoked.

The art and journaling were therapeutic to look back on after I was discharged. It was then I realized my artwork and written record were a prayer of thanksgiving. They represented the gratitude that had filled my chest and discharged tension I hadn't known I was holding.

I hadn't wanted to forget the significance and my awareness of being held.

~

**Whose Hands Held Me?**
*(journaled July 30, 2020)*

Firm pressure held and comforted me while in a frazzled state I'd climbed up onto that stainless steel surgical table.

"Would you like a pillow?" someone asked.

I'd pursed my lips and nodded as I adjusted myself into what comfort I could find. Belly down on the hard, icy surface I lay. With elbows out, like the flapping wings of a threatened turkey, I'd instinctively known I didn't want to be the featured star of a celebratory meal. The backs of my fingertips cradled my bony chin. The pillow I'd been offered helped support and relax my neck, rolled to the left and facing the radiologist.

Cheek to pillow, I could now see where the radiologist stood, as well as the someone—a technician perhaps—who'd offered me the pillow. To my immediate left, the radiologist's hands initially prepared the site on my back with sterile gloved hands and a cleaning solution to reduce the risk of infection before inserting the central venous line.

The contrast dye, I imagined, was coursing through my arteries to assist the radiologist's steady hand. This, as he inserted the long, empty syringe between the vertebrae.

Without a mirror, I'd used my sense of touch to record details. I felt one hand on my lower back, then another.

Who's hands? Whose reassuring hands held me? The radiologists, I'd first believed. They were not. No other individual was at my side holding me. Of this I was certain, yet I could feel steading hands on my low back.

Awake and conscious during the procedure, the radiologist moved slightly to where he then stood staring intently at a monitor. As he prepared, I could see both his hands. Whose hands then held me with compassionate, downward pressure with precision stillness? There was abundant evidence of hands holding me. What evidence? I sensed it, felt it, and those hands immobilized automatic thoughts and replaced them with peace and serenity.

Freed from anxious thoughts, the dread had lifted. A humpback's powerful fluke enabled its massive bulk to lift and leap from the ocean's depths and darkness, breach the surface, and embrace the light.

Prayers had been lifted. Of this I was certain. Fear had vanished while I was held. Those firm, gentle hands must have been His, the Holy Spirit.

Under His protection, I was at peace and without pain. throughout the spinal tap.

Gentle Jesus-Thank you.

The radiologist had radiated calm, and with a single minded purpose exuded confidence. He'd unexpectedly spoken aloud. From the corner of my eye, with head turned and cheek inscribed into a dense hospital pillow, I'd watched. And listened with curiosity.

To whom he spoke, I was uncertain.

Maybe me? I didn't think so but had been grateful that he'd provided a running commentary. Who else watched? Were others viewing and learning while I was unaware? I found it helpful to know what to expect as he outlined the procedure step by step aloud.

"I'm aiming for the sweet spot between the vertebrae."

My mind was without fear. Thoughts didn't race. I was held.

With gratitude I'd given thanks:

*Thank you, Lord, for giving the specialist clarity, focus, a gifted mind, intellectual curiosity, a love of medicine and science and the wisdom to discern with perfect precision his work. Thank you for ensuring his eyes, heart, and mind are in perfect unison. All for me.*

*Thank you for making me unique, just as I am. For my mind, body, intellect, and*

> creativity. For compassionate relationships that lift me, a loving family, and communities of care. Thank you, Lord, for giving me a little faith, and a desire for more.
> Amen.

~

Afterwards, there had been an *aha*. Light shone through distortions for an interval of discernment. Fluoroscopy and prayer, I realized, were only two viable tools, which I could use to journey towards wellness. There could be others, I hadn't yet explored. With this *aha* came a bonus realization—a spark of meta-cognition.

There'd been a renewed flame of hope ignited.

During the hospital admission between July 24–29, I was able to reimagine myself as child-like, curious, beloved, held, safe, and protected.

That spark of hope made a difference. I wanted to take care of myself. Desired to feel and express my needs. I acknowledged I needed help.

In short, I hadn't prioritized myself, was stuck and frozen by fear. I'd become this lost soul who meticulously detailed physical symptoms through the lenses of loss, grief, and illness.

I was bogged down and firmly entrenched in the mire.

I hadn't thought to ask about underlying causes of my challenging physical symptoms. Those symptoms I'd experienced throughout and up until the summer of 2020. I hadn't realized these same symptoms could be related to early developmental perspective and/or adverse childhood experiences. There hadn't been that necessary someone special to help comfort, support, and guide me to understand how my childhood had informed my core beliefs, underlying assumptions, and automatic thoughts.

Our parents, Sandra's and mine, hadn't been capable to comfort or support us or to help me see through a proactive mental health lens a restorative action plan. Mom had been too busy with her own distorted thoughts and the provision of what she deemed more pressing needs. She had a laser focus on our physical health and wellness. She expertly provided shelter, nutrition, and physical safety. Dad had abandoned and neglected to shoulder any responsibility at all.

I hadn't realized the value then of speaking about fear and mental anguish, or the importance of testing out ways to strategize when I experienced distorted thoughts. Stress constantly triggered an anxious heart and mind, which in an elevated state of hyper-arousal, feared.

Meanwhile, I dreaded, but waited in desperate anticipation for each successive investigation. I desperately needed clarity and answers. I continued to hold onto hope that complex physical symptoms I experienced would provide necessary data. Information that medical specialists could interpret successfully. If only there'd been the necessary just-right specialist, who could knowingly interpret what the vast collection of data hadn't yet revealed – a diagnosis.

*I shoulda coulda woulda asked for help, but didn't.*

I was strong, yet weak and ignorant of the fact that my basic childhood needs for love and attachment hadn't been met. Had they been I might have had the resilience to speak up and ask for help I not only required but deserved.

The sheer physical effort to control anger, hostility and regret while attempting to survive distorted thoughts caused dysregulation and exacerbated fears. Worries exacted a heavy cost as my body continued to keep score.

JOCELYN BYSTROM

# CHAPTER FIFTEEN

### Struggling with Indecision

E arly on a Monday the first week of August 2020, I crept out of our bedroom while Dale slept. I headed outside to the back deck to delight in the sunrise and record the dream which had awakened me.

Under blankets in a comfy recliner, I closed my eyes and listened to birds chittering and vocalizing morning delight. I luxuriated in the pleasurable caress of a gentle breeze on my face, the only skin uncovered and not protected by blankets. Wide awake, my senses were alert. I pulled out my journal and made a detailed record of what I'd dreamed:

Fractured thoughts and billowing, twisted clouds danced across the landscape, a funnel cloud during a summer storm. Then, lightning struck abruptly, and flashes of brilliance illuminated the darkened sky. The lightening awakened a dreamer who danced across my imagination. Believing the climax of the storm was imminent, and that funnel clouds would touch down shortly, igniting a tornado, the dancer painted a crescendo of sound across the sky, increasing in force like the flight of a wounded bumblebee.

The principal dancer's performance intensified, then calmed. Unaccompanied, she danced like the Aurora Borealis, with curtains of colored light across the glowing night sky. She told a compelling story as she pointed graceful arms and hands and reached and placed twinkling lights across the heavens.

Then, with the intensity of a whip cracking, a second blinding flash darted across the sky. Twinkle lights vanished as the music reached a crescendo, and a funnel cloud touched down, enflaming the now swirling ballerina into a whipped throw. She executed a fouetté, and in doing so, became the Black Swan, performing a seemingly never-ending amount of turns before being transformed herself into a spinning tornado.

In the storm's aftermath, fissures had been torn across the darkened, starless stage. The music was silenced. Unlike gold and silver refined by fire, the dancer lay transformed. Bereft of music and soul without technical skills or artistic maturity. Her body sprawled like a broken bird.

~

Between August 3–16, my cell phone rang repeatedly as I continued to seek help with piercing headaches which were an easy eight on a zero to ten pain scale. Headaches which were now present upon waking lasted hours and incapacitated me. Were my headaches the result of the lumbar puncture procedure? I'd read in an article that spinal headaches were a common complication since the spinal tap procedure required a puncture of the tough membrane that surrounds the spinal cord and, in the lower spine, the lumbar and sacral nerve roots.

A highly specialized team of medical practitioners had formed over the years and as of August 1, included a neuro-stroke specialist. I had my first consult with the most recent addition to my team from the VGH (Vancouver General Hospital) Stroke Program. He referred me back to the Comox Valley Hospital for an additional highly specialized MRI, marked URGENT.

*What now?*

Although the results of this MRI showed little of significance, the neuro-stroke specialist was reassured by what he *hadn't* seen. With still no clarity, the flurry of calls continued between myself and specialists and the ever-expanding group who now collaborated on my care.

~

Our family camping trip planned for months would be a go. It would also be a much-needed interval, full of the anticipated deliciousness of corned beef, sauerkraut, and Swiss cheese between slices of toasted rye bread. There would be a period of rest to enjoy our adult children, their partners, our cousins, and nephew, between caregiving and yet another hospital admission. This time I'd be headed back to Vancouver General on the BC coast's mainland from Vancouver Island and my home in Comox.

Desperate to find a caregiver to cover Mom's care Thursday night through Sunday when Dale would arrive back home solo after escorting me to Vancouver for this next emergency neurology admission, I phoned my friend Cindy long-distance. I'd already tried everyone I could think of locally and come up with nil. Even though our dear friend would need to travel to help us out, I asked. Thankfully, Cindy's forthcoming yes delighted demoralized eardrums. Without hesitation, she offered to fly directly to Comox in time for Dale and I to leave for the family camp out on Aug 20. We'd be able to celebrate Kristen's birthday after all. I booked Cindy a flight on Harbour Air and hoped the stars would align.

That Sunday night, my epileptologist called. She explained that a collaborative decision had been made to admit me to the neurology ward at VGH, and she'd arranged that I would be admitted the following morning, Monday, August 17. Instantly, I'd burst into tears, remembering the plans we had to celebrate Kristen's birthday at the family camp out leaving Thursday. I'd needed to make the reservations months earlier to secure a group site. And now ... *this?* There was no way I'd be able to leave for the trip.

Instead of being delighted that clarity and potential relief from the massive headaches I now suffered, and that help was now finally being offered, I was overwhelmed. Overcome by the intense rush of emotion as I considered a planned emergency admission. The result of which impacted skewed priorities.

What I did next shocked even me. Rather than being conquered by tears and thoughts which would have taken me to darker depths, I spoke up.

I dared to ask for what I needed.

"Can it wait till next Monday?" Then, anxiously, I awaited an answer.

What prompted me to ask? Desperation. I'd lost so much and couldn't bear more. Perhaps it was my soul's cry for help. A spark of hope had flickered, then threatened to be extinguished.

Would anyone ever understand or be able to tell me what was going on in my obviously complex body? Many brilliant minds seemed baffled.

During what seemed a forever pause, but was probably only seconds, I listened.

"Perhaps we could make that work," my epileptologist said. "I'll see what I can figure out . . . and get back to you." Stunned by her progressive and respectful attitude, I thanked her and hung up.

Dale suggested I not expect a second call that same day, knowing I had high hopes and did not want me to be disappointed. But bless her heart. She called back shortly to say she'd had success.

"It's a go and has been agreed upon by all concerned." In that instant, I knew she cared deeply. How often I wondered, after hearing this, do specialists work endless hours on weekends and evenings without gratitude, labouring while we're unaware?

"Thank you, thank you, thank you!" escaped my lips, giving birth to my dimpled cheeks. "Dale, it's arranged. I'll be admitted Monday morning, August 24."

Hallelujah!

~

As I packed, for the camping trip and subsequent admission August 19, my tank was empty, but my heart full. The admission would include a prolonged seventy-two-hour EEG with video surveillance. An electroencephalogram technologist would monitor my brain's activity at the bedside around the clock. My epileptologist had fierce determination. She worked diligently to locate the secret key and unlock Pandora's box. She cared for and about me. She appeared to be a Type A overachiever just like someone else I know, predisposed with a tendency toward workaholism. I hoped she had a better approach to work-life balance than I; however, I was incredibly grateful for her passionate devotion to her work and expertise. I'd been constantly reassured knowing she was thorough.

She investigated with an exhaustive pursuit, rather than simply the five W's: who, what, why, when, and how?

Who might she collaborate with that could help contribute the missing piece? What caused the abnormal epileptiform discharges with spiked peaks on each of my previous EEGs? Why would an epileptologist be taking such a keen interest in my care, if I didn't have epilepsy? Had she not sufficient data yet to determine whether I had a form of epilepsy caused by a brain tumor, stroke, traumatic brain injury, or an infection of the central nervous system?

When would medical practitioners be ready to give me a clear diagnosis and much-needed clarity? How could an epileptologist accomplish what seemed impossible?

If anyone could figure out a diagnosis, I knew it would be Dr. Percy. My epileptologist provided respectful expertise and so much more. Our therapeutic relationship facilitated my desire for wellness, and she'd adapted her expertise and treatment to my unique needs by eliciting and responding to feedback. She'd asked, but I hadn't trusted easily then.

She'd managed my strong emotions, and, on each occasion—whether it was in person, on the phone, or at the hospital bedside during admissions at VGH—we spoke. She worked collaboratively by recruiting a top-notch team of professionals with big-picture thinking.

I appreciated that she took the lead and that

she prioritized her availability to respond when I was overwhelmed. Dr. Percy was a leader of leaders, and masterful advocate for my health and wellness, while I was sliding down a slippery slope. I felt blessed.

~

Strangely enough, the anticipation of leaving Comox excited me amidst lockdowns, as the Canadian and British Columbia governments enforced ever-stricter public health safety measures aimed to flatten the curve. I was headed on a holiday of sorts eight months into a global pandemic, despite the trip being caused by complex ill-health.

How weird was it that I considered medical investigation a holiday?

~

Dale and I had cancelled all weekend and holiday plans other than our much-anticipated summer getaway after Mom moved in months earlier. She could no longer be safely left alone. By May, in desperation, I had left her on her own viewing a curling game for my sanity more frequently than I cared to admit.

Chosen moments for sanity inscribed shame.

I longed for any opportunity to remove myself from the responsibility that is caregiving. Even if only for a day. It had been eight months since news of a deadly virus reached us, and I'd read online I wasn't alone as I fantasized. Citizens of the world hoped for what seemed impossible during a global pandemic—a vacation.

While others prayed for a vaccine and cure, I wanted more than a few hours to myself. The responsibility of caregiving was both a labour of love and darned hard work. I had the heart for it; but it was an emotional burden during a pandemic. Being a care-partner is a lonely road, especially before you seek help, believing naively that you can manage on your own. When I was finally ready to locate the care I desperately needed for Mom, it wasn't available during the pandemic. There was no access to adult day-programs for family members with dementia and/or bathing care for Mom.

An excerpt from my journal speaks to my apprehension that first time I'd needed to bathe my mother:

> *I wonder if I can do this.* I'd hoped never to need to. Here I am, here goes. Mom's in the bathroom, and for the first time the door is not locked. After preparing the upstairs bathroom with what I thought would be necessary and Mom might want, I left. I'd paced outside the door, left open just a crack, enough that I could peek in, or help if she had a fall. This seemed like a good idea, common sense.
>
> I could hear her slowly undressing and was surprised how long it took. I imagined her balancing on one leg and lifting the other while taking off her pants. Then I peeked. She was seated on the toilet, undressing. My sweet, reserved mother guarded her privacy for as long as I can remember. I had never seen her naked and if the truth be told, didn't want to.
>
> Certainly, this can't be what she wants either. My heart was racing, and I wasn't the one getting undressed. I know that she's as anxious as I am.
>
> I left Mom an assortment of towels and the bath chair I'd positioned in the tub for her safety. I'd bought it for her years ago and purchased it after finding an old fashioned stacking stool with its hairpin aluminum legs and vinyl covered seat in her apartment's bathtub.
>
> Later, when I'd moved her out of her apartment and into our home last March, I'd found and rescued it from her storage locker beside the Christmas decorations. She'd

forgotten where it was, and that she'd been gifted it.

Next, I reminded Mom that when she was ready to get into the tub to use the grab rails, which Dale had installed for me the previous year as my balance began to get shaky. I reminded her that she should use them to get into the tub and then turn to sit facing the shower and tap. I suggested she might cover up with a large hand towel knowing how modest she was and that her being uncovered wasn't an option.

I waited anxiously and heard Mom continue to undress as I paced back and forth in the hallway like a trapped lioness at the zoo. Up and down the short hallway, I strode. From the kitchen to my bedroom and back, I continued to pace before daring to peek in, again. I couldn't stand still. Nervousness kept me moving. I didn't want to hover and embarrass her. Finally, I heard the shower curtain pull across the metal rod with a scrape and she said, "Okay."

I headed in and reached around the curtain at the end closest to the taps and hand shower wand which I'd left hanging. I turned on the taps and water fell into the tub as I adjusted its temperature, speaking to her all the while to reassure and calm her, I thought. I purposefully used my calming mom's and teacher's voice. A voice that this empty nester mom and teacher on medical leave hadn't practiced for quite a while.

Mom was shocked by the sudden rush of water as it burst out of the shower head. She jumped instinctively, thinking the water was hotter than she could manage. I'd previously made sure it was only lukewarm and dipped my wiggling fingers into the flow.

I attempted to redirect her thoughts by handing her the shower head and suggesting she point it at her toes to check the temperature. I thought if she had control, she might not be as anxious.

She didn't seem to know what I'd meant as I reached to touch her toes and give her a visual example. I realized in that moment that she didn't and couldn't remember the labels or words for her various body parts. That had been a significant realization. As I moved around the curtain from one side to the other in a discombobulated shower dance to respect her privacy, I made an awkward first attempt to bathe my mom.

Was this my mother? It was, though I wished it wasn't.

When we'd agreed that the water temperature was just right, I'd taken the wand and aimed the water away from her feet.

Then as I showered her legs below the knees and ever so slowly up her legs. "How does that feel, Mom?" I asked. This, as I prepared to slide to the other end of the curtain and transfer the wand so I could wash her hair. I touched each body part gently, then named it. I started with "shoulder," and brought the warmed water to that spot as my other hand caressed with soap.

All the while, Mom clung to the hand towel, shielding herself from my eyes and her embarrassment. Like a nun, I attempted to avert my eyes downward. I fumbled along inadequately and shampooed and rinsed her short grey hair.

For the past several months, I'd taken her once a week to her hair salon, where she'd been having her hair cut for over twenty years. But this got expensive and was no longer an option due to the pandemic and her deteriorating condition. While rinsing her hair, I'd been reminded of the Winnie the Pooh visor I'd used for Keith as a child to keep shampoo out of his eyes. It would have been handy now, I thought with a smile. After rinsing and washing Mom's back, I'd had enough. It isn't easy to bathe your mother. With a gentle touch, so as not to scare her, I stroked her hand, then offered her the soap, saying, "I'm going to leave you on your own now and give you some privacy to wash your private parts." Had I just said that to my mother? I fled to the hallway where I lingered and wondered with apprehension if she needed help to get out of the tub.

It's begun. I am now officially my mom's full time caregiver, I realized.

~

Dale and I recognized we needed a break, shortly after Mom's first Jocelyn-assisted bath. Time for the two of us. And hours to do those mundane or spontaneous things couples enjoy. We hadn't been able to make plans for ourselves for months and everyone everywhere was missing face-to-face interactions outside their homes. I longed to visit a friend, go for a bike ride on our new e-bicycles, or to go anywhere. With self-pity and in isolation, I was oblivious that the world was waiting for connection and community too. I wasn't alone in that.

Public health care had offered one four-hour respite block each week back in June as Mom's care needs escalated. It was only after I ended up in the hospital at the end of July and had met with social workers that respite care was increased to three four-hour blocks each week. My overwhelmed state had been noted. I wasn't managing.

By the end of August, due to the increased demand for respite care during the pandemic, I lost one block of the respite care. I couldn't manage with just eight hours. Perhaps if I'd been well enough to have ventured outside or past our back deck, I might have had my caregiving batteries rejuvenated enough. I had gratitude for the respite I received but needed more.

~

I made a list of what to pack, as well as what was needed to be organized for Mom, as I prepared for our August 20 departure. With the precision of a pilot making final preparations for a safe takeoff or landing, I methodically checked off items.

I purchased groceries for our friend Cindy, who'd be arriving shortly. I created a notebook filled with instructions and routines detailing everything I did daily. She hadn't needed these and was a more than capable care-partner. It was I who had needed to make lists, triple-check each itemized list and to ensure everything needed was indeed ready. I also had to be certain my suitcase was ready for my hospital admission, in addition to my backpack, which would double as an overnight bag for both the family campout and my subsequent three-day stay at Vancouver General Hospital's neurology ward.

Extra masks, gloves, and hand sanitizer to protect against COVID-19 were necessities. Items I'd need to protect myself from the virus as I headed to the ferry and then onward to Vancouver General Hospital on my own. For months now, I'd travelled under provincial public health guidelines and restrictions for essential travel. Constraints which impeded travel between health regions in British Columbia. Restrictions, which by this date were common across Canada. Residents of Vancouver Island could only go to the mainland for essential travel or medical reasons.

When I travelled independently, I worried constantly that I'd pick up the virus while in transit. Masks were mandatory on BC Ferries, yet no one policed the requirements or restrictions. I couldn't be sure the person standing or seated next to me stayed at the recommended six feet distance, or in Canada, the length of a hockey stick.

Lineups being what they were plus human nature made travellers want to get where they were going quickly and to return home safely. Self-absorbed egos often were resentful, or non-compliant of stickers recently placed on floor tiles reminding folks they were required to stand in line two metres apart.

At the height of infection, when positive test results of the then dreaded SARS-CoV-2, variant of coronavirus that caused COVID-19, were growing exponentially, there were still only forty-six cases in the province of British Columbia, Canada, and none in Comox, on Vancouver Island where I live.

It wasn't until March 11, 2020, that positive test results were confirmed on Vancouver Island. In grocery stores, public restrooms, or for essential services like BC Ferries, where walk-on passengers queued to board and disembark, inevitably, there was an unavoidable crush.

I'd felt safe in the Comox Valley. But after March 11, I had only a little courage and wanted more. I had a little faith and needed more.

As I became more incapacitated in late-July, I needed a medical escort each time I made a trip to Vancouver. In the days leading up to my August admission to VGH's neurology ward I'd still paid bills, filed for reimbursement through Mom's health insurance provider for her incurred expenses, sent necessary medical forms to doctors and specialists for me, and filed required paperwork to update my medical leave from teaching.

Paperwork—ours and Mom's—overwhelmed me. Some took precedence and other bills and forms were left piling up on the back burner. Mom's annual income tax paperwork had been due April 30 and was still incomplete. I'd been anxious about this and then the deadline had been extended due to the pandemic first till June 1, and then later to another date. I'd lost track and then forgot altogether what I'd needed to gather for Mom, where her papers had been stored after I'd moved her out of her apartment several months earlier and where now they might be. I would get them done ASAHP—as soon as *humanly* possible.

Dale often needed to take time off work in his new and ever-expanded role as care-partner. This besides staying home with Mom in my absence. It took a toll that I was often unaware of as he silenced his own fears and medicated his pain. We hadn't wanted a string of potentially virus-carrying care-partners in our home, anyway. And as Plans A, B, C, and D fell through and repetitive pleas for respite seemed to fall on deaf ears, it got harder to ask. We stopped asking.

In my mind, it had become vitally important to assure Mom was cared for each time I prepared to leave Comox. If not me, then who? Who would take on all mom's routines, tasks, and details? I now parented my mother with lies of omission. Perhaps later I'd have the wherewithal to explain, and we'd both understand. Perhaps not.

~

The afternoon of August 20, Dale and I picked up our friend and Mom's caregiver Cindy, who'd flown in by seaplane on Harbour Air. We were headed home from the Comox marina's seaplane base when we were unexpectedly rear-ended.

The collision was an intense shock. My eyes had been closed, as I was feeling unwell and had a major headache. I'd been leaning back in the passenger seat, head against the headrest, when we were hit from behind.

Dale, astute and observant, had slammed on the brakes and come to a full stop just shy of the car in front who'd stopped without warning. He'd hit his brakes at the last moment after he'd noticed a pedestrian stepping out into the crosswalk at the last moment. The driver behind us had not. We were sandwiched by the impact, first from behind and then again as we jetted forward and collided. Dale, Cindy, and I each sustained back and neck injuries. Dale additionally injured his knees.

Not a great precursor to our planned early evening departure and four-hour long drive to the family campout, but I wouldn't let it stop us.

After Dale dealt with ICBC (Insurance Corporation of British Columbia) regarding the accident, we waved to Mom and Cindy and headed out for camp at Rathtrevor Provincial Park.

"Have a wonderful trip." Mom said, as she waved late in the evening of August 20th, and then blew me a kiss.

~

The campout had been a wonderful respite. I arrived in Vancouver August 23.

I'd been grateful to arrive at Rory and Cindy's house, after my nephew Jean-Luc, who'd come to Vancouver Island with Kristen and her boyfriend Matt to camp with us, accompanied me on BC Ferries as we'd headed to Vancouver from camp.

Reaching their home, I headed to bed for a nap. Happily, ensconced in what came to be affectionately known as *my room*, at my home away from home in Vancouver. I visited with Rory after napping, then stayed up way too late enjoying the freedom and respite on what felt like a mini-vacation. Late, far past my usual 10 p.m. bedtime, I fell exhausted into bed after adding distilled water to my continuous positive airway pressure machine (CPAP) tank and donning the nasal mask. But despite the lateness of the hour, I lay awake with an anxious, busy brain too super-charged to rest.

Usually used for obstructive apnea, my CPAP was used to help regulate sleep and possibly reduce the frequency and intensity of severe migraine-like headaches I experienced.

Dale and I both now used CPAP machines, side by side at night while we slept. I hoped it would help reduce my debilitating headaches, which left me wilted and with irregular sleep hygiene.

I was told to bring enough things to the neurology ward to entertain myself for three days without getting out of bed, since I would be attached to the EEG electrodes for the duration of my admission. I'd brought my CPAP machine, laptop, sketchbook, scissors, markers, and magazines to read, and then later collage with selected images used in my art therapy classes. I'm a creative type and hadn't wanted to binge Netflix for three days straight. There'd been no restrictions listed in the pre-admission packet, so I packed what I thought I needed and wanted.

The following day, August 24, I was grateful to be dropped off at the hospital's front doors after lunch. I entered alone, as no support person or family members were allowed to accompany you during Stage One pandemic protocols, measures that were being strictly enforced at every entrance.

One admissions volunteer commented on the size of my international-sized suitcase as I entered the building, and her remarks hadn't been kind.

"Looks like you expect it'll be a vacation!" Then under her breath, when she thought I was out of earshot, she added, "Some people are so entitled, and bloody high-maintenance."

I wanted to defend my choices and explain but did not waste my breath. Some people are just plain ignorant as to how their words wound.

I needed to use the Q-TIP strategy and to: Quit Taking It Personally—a helpful distress tolerance tool I'd learned years earlier when I'd needed the thickened skin of a rhinoceros to protect my vulnerable heart. I reminded myself to check the facts. The comment had been about her, not me. Regardless, it still wounded me in my state of anxiousness about the next three days of neurological investigations.

That evening I had visits from various specialists and answered questions asked by various fellows, undergoing supervised, sub-specialty medical training, in both neurology and psychiatry, prior to when the EEG technician appeared at my door.

He'd come to attach the essential components of an EEG machine including electrodes, amplifiers, a computer control module, and a display device to my scalp. There would be a technician monitoring the display for the next three days, or so I was told.

The following day, my first full day at the neurology ward, was filled with diagnostic testing to assess how different medications affected my brain and body. Exhausted after a long day of assessment, I fell asleep more easily on night two, despite the electrodes glued to my scalp and a braid of trailing wires. Transmitting, I hoped, what my voice had silenced.

Upon waking the morning of Wednesday, August 26, I was told I was being sent home after forty hours of analysis rather than the three full days of assessment I'd expected and been prepared to stay. I was discharged from my bed with its padded rails to protect flailing limbs and my head from concussion, and specialized, crinkly plastic pads to protect the mattress and bedding from a bladder that might empty unexpectedly were I to have a seizure.

I'd been monitored twenty-four seven by video surveillance, intravenously given new medications as a technician sat by my bedside monitoring my brain for abnormal readings, and told I could expect seizures. After all, there had been repeated EEGs between 2013–2020, most of which recorded abnormal results neurologists seemed concerned about.

Dale and I had been told to arrange for my release Friday, but now the discharge nurse said only, "Doctors have taken you off Wellbutrin to determine whether it is the underlying cause of the spells and side effects you've reported."

Earlier I had described headaches that never dulled, concentrated on the left side of my forehead above my left eye. I'd reported notable changes in my cognition, poor concentration, and that my ability to focus between reading one line of text and the next proved difficult. I experienced immense fatigue from prolonged reading, and headaches after just fifteen minutes of any form of concentrated cognitive effort. The doctor who'd discharged me, Dr. Thiessen, a name I'd only remembered because I'd recorded it in my health journal, had exited the private room in the neurology ward the previous evening after making rounds with essentially the same minimal information.

"We'll want to know whether the Wellbutrin, which we've taken you off of, changes the frequency and/or intensity of your myoclonic jerks." The nurse continued. I'd thought Dr. Thiessen would be back, or that I'd see my neurologist again before being discharged. It seemed only hours earlier I'd been at this same desk being admitted.

With my re-packed suitcase and backpack, I listened to the attending discharge nurse quash my hopes for clarity, rush me from a needed bed, as she read the discharge papers aloud. It seemed she was in a hurry and dutifully reporting what was required to ensure that I would adopt and implement the instructions written without any further elaboration. She then asked, "Do you have any additional questions?" Overwhelmed, I had many and asked none.

I believed they were questions she couldn't answer, so why bother? I tucked the all-important discharge papers into my backpack for safekeeping along with my wallet. I shouldered my backpack, grabbed the handle of my suitcase, and headed toward the elevator. Alone.

My suitcase thankfully had wheels. I also carried a large, white, plastic hospital bag. You know, the one everyone gets when they head home from the hospital—white with large lettering that says patient belongings, name and room number written on the side? It had been a parting gift, for all the items that hadn't fit back into my suitcase, including dirty laundry, bedding brought from home knowing it was a necessity for a comfortable night's sleep, and the warm jacket I hadn't needed in August, but that could double as a blanket, or rain jacket, if required. It can be incredibly windy on BC Ferries, especially as a walk-on passenger travelling without the shelter of a car. I'd needed these creature comforts despite their weight. Altogether, my accoutrements were more than I could manage. I naively expected there would be someone there to help.

I arranged for our daughter, Kristen, to pick me up shortly after I learned that I was being discharged. She quickly decided to leave her home office, where she'd been working remotely since the beginning of the global pandemic. She dropped everything to come, but the waiting seemed an eternity as I sat overwhelmed and alone with my thoughts, unanswered questions, and belongings.

Why was I going home so soon? I didn't get it. My discharge papers, which I read and reread while I waited had minimal information except for a new medication regime. Dr. Percy had reassured me I wouldn't be discharged unless someone could be with me. I needed someone due to my reduced ability to concentrate and remember details. I'd counted on having a trusted individual who could listen and remember any additional, unwritten discharge instructions, and make a record of what the neurology team had discovered, as well as plans for moving forward.

None of this happened.

~

Kristen texted: *I'm here.* She was able to park close by in a special zone for patient drop-off and pick-up but could not come into the hospital itself due to COVID-19 protocols. I collected and balanced as much as possible on top of my suitcase with wheels and carried the rest to the arranged meeting place. I was spent when at last I saw her smiling face and outstretched arms, ready to help.

On route back to Burnaby, we scouted for a pharmacy to pick up two new medications I was prescribed on discharge. My plan was to stay overnight at Kristen's while I made arrangements to travel home earlier than expected. I phoned and reserved a seat on the connecting Island Link, back to Courtenay, where Dale would leave Mom briefly with our neighbour keeping an eye on her, to pick me up.

Kristen stopped at an unfamiliar pharmacy for convenience. The discharge nurse indicated I needed to continue with the new medications I'd been given at the hospital, so rather than waiting we hung out while the prescriptions were filled.

Meanwhile, I attempted to answers Kristen's questions about the hospital admission; however, I mostly apologized for my inability to remember details. Thankfully, she listened and allowed me to vent. And, in doing so, reassured me. I was incredibly grateful for her compassion in my weakness. I unpacked my fears and emotions until it was time to check back in at the pharmacy. Then with new medications in hand, we headed straight home to Kristen's basement suite in Burnaby.

I was on the phone most of the day making travel arrangements and re-packing for the return trip. It had been an unbelievable holiday, and one which would most certainly not get a five-star Yelp review.

After supper, I opened the pharmacy bag containing the two newly labelled medications, which I was to take with food, at dinner time. I took what I needed out of each pill bottle, and with a full water bottle swallowed the exact prescribed quantities recommended during discharge.

Later I felt odd and couldn't quite explain the feeling. Curious, I took out the plastic pill bottles and more carefully read the labels. Had I mistaken the correct dosages, believing I'd remembered correctly? I put on my reading glasses and prepared to reread the labels, with the clarity of my reading glasses, rather than my progressives. Some of the new medications have such tiny writing on them, it seems almost like they don't expect you to read the fine print. More carefully this time, I read the entire label . . . and then stared at the top line.

It was then I realized with horror that I had taken the correct amounts, but of *someone else's* medication. Unbeknownst to me, I had taken a stranger's medications. Kristen immediately phoned the pharmacy to inquire what had happened, and to immediately learn if I was in danger. I feared she'd need to drive me back to the ER, not knowing what I'd accidentally ingested. Elevated anxiety ensured I couldn't think straight.

Clear-minded, I knew I would have had the required discernment to prevent what had just happened. My mind froze, and then fled all over the map, as I fought off catastrophic thoughts, and imagined dangerous drug interactions. What had I taken? I needed to know.

Kristen handled the whole situation with the same calm Dale demonstrates when my anxiety skyrockets. After an urgent call to the pharmacy, she spoke to an extremely embarrassed and apologetic pharmacist, who after learning of my current medications, and what I'd accidentally taken, believed that there would be no need to return to Emergency. He explained to Kristen that I would most likely just sleep off the medication, with no harmful or dangerous drug interactions, or side effects. He reiterated, more than once, that he didn't believe we needed to return to the Emergency Department, and in my sleepy, overwhelmed state, I wanted to trust this advice. Most of all I didn't want to go back to the hospital. More importantly, I trusted Kristen, who is wise beyond her years. I trusted her with my life. Eventually I slept.

It turned out I'd ingested someone else's prescribed medical marijuana, in addition to their heart medication. Some days, I believe you just need to fall asleep trusting that your prayers will be answered, and that your needs are covered. Simply too tired to think any further about this exhausting day, Kristen hugged me, and I closed my eyes to recharge.

Kristen monitored me through the night, as upon reflection I'm certain she feared an event we hadn't bargained for. I had feared loss of self-control for nearly five decades and purposefully chosen to not experiment with smoking or recreational drugs. Now, I knew the feeling: of being powerless, unable to make sound judgements, or communicate my needs effectively. My fears were confirmed; I'm not a fan of giving up control.

~

My epileptologist, Dr. Percy, later told me that a post-admission EEG reported no change, and those abnormal discharges were still occurring and between one-half to eight seconds in length. I concluded that it wasn't the anti-anxiety Wellbutrin that had caused the unusual epileptiform discharges. What then, was causing the multitude of physical, cognitive, and emotional symptoms I'd been experiencing all along? Symptoms which continued to increase each month in frequency, intensity, and duration.

The remaining days in August I spent sitting, reclining, or sleeping.

~

September arrived and with it a cold, bleak season of prolonged waiting for diagnostic clarity, caregiving for my mother, and worrying towards wellness.

I became so very weary and spent entire days dozing and sleeping. I struggled to maintain a regular relaxed breathing pattern. Dale noted and commented one night about my shallow breathing as we lay in bed. He'd been reading as I dozed when I realized my breaths were more than shallow. At times, there were gaps when I didn't breathe. A few days later, in similar circumstances, I'd blacked out and was unconscious.

I couldn't remember what happened after I'd struggled for breath. When I came to, I didn't know how long I'd been out.

"How long was I unconscious?" I asked Dale. He looked puzzled, as if I'd awakened from a bad dream, and responded, "I thought you'd fallen asleep."

Many lifted me in prayer at a time I couldn't pray for my own needs. I simply longed to be held, needed and capable again. Nothing made sense.

I required more emotional support that ever as I continued to be saturated with heaviness, the burden of caregiving, and struggled with indecision. To put Mom in care, or not? That was the over-arching question with which I battled. I wore too many varied hats and hadn't enjoyed wearing any hat my whole life.

Care partner, caregiver, and care recipient were only three of the hats I wore simultaneously. Woman of Faith, wife, mother, daughter, and teacher, my most precious headpieces had been stripped away. Forms to prioritize Mom's placement in a care facility, due to the intolerable risk to my health and wellbeing were waiting on my desk. And, had been for months. It was time.

I signed on the dotted line to place Mom in care.

# CHAPTER SIXTEEN

## Speaking My Truth

Like a hummingbird, my mind darted without slowing or sitting. I accelerated rather than stopping to take the time to perch or recharge. Territorial, I darted here and there, chasing away fear with pinpoint maneuverability.

I didn't trust easily and couldn't risk my heart. I believed in Dale's integrity and strength despite not conveying my trust in him convincingly. My distrustful disposition hadn't changed since I was a child when I hadn't truly believed I was enough and unmet emotional needs spoke volumes.

There'd been yet another trip to the mainland, and Vancouver General Hospital, to meet with my epileptologist in late September. On October 1, I had an appointment with another neurological specialist. I sat in Comox staring at my laptop monitor, in a virtual waiting room, for a Zoom appointment with my newest doc. who specialized in sleep disorders. He referred me for a two-day overnight sleep study since I continued to have trouble breathing at night and didn't feel well-rested upon waking. I inhaled shallow breaths with insufficient air as I worried myself to sleep each night while I awaited the sleep assessment. The assessment was on hold due to the pandemic and wasn't scheduled for the foreseeable future. Each night as I fell asleep intense migraine-like headaches at the base of my left temporal lobe created pain and caused sleeplessness, despite taking medication to resolve the headaches. Sleep managed to elude its pursuer and escaped into the night.

~

Even after I'd experienced the hot-stroke protocol and six-day hospitalization in July 2020, and three-day neurological investigation in late August, I'd waited for a correct diagnosis. For goodness' sake, it was October now . . . and the waiting hadn't ended. Once again, the temperatures dropped, leaves had fallen, and winter storms threatened.

~

Fierce musical notes showed up as intense seizures and shortness of breath. Harsh discordant sounds suggested terrorized screams may have become a reality. But, without a brave space, I hadn't allowed them to materialize. With disharmonious chords I'd wept in the shower, my safe place to permit tears. No one must know how weak I was.

My voice had been strategically silenced by a strong-willed inner child, like Tchaikovsky's "1812 Overture" with its intended syncopated cannons. The climactic volley of cannon fire Tchaikovsky would later write into his composition in 1880 to commemorate the successful Russian defense against Napoleon's invading armies, wasn't added until 1954. I hadn't needed to wait seventy-four years, but even six at this point seemed too long. Through September and the first weeks of October 2020, I sketched and journaled using Dr. Ira Progoff's Intensive Journal Process (IJP).

~

*Always tell the truth.* Momma taught me: "If you can't say anything nice, don't say anything at all." I didn't have the courage to add another layer of conflict to already super-charged emotions. So, I said, nothing.

I completed a series of integrated writing exercises and prompts during the IJP workshops and recorded reflections about different areas of my life (i.e., personal relationships, body and health, life history, dreams and imagery, and the meaning in life, etc.). Each prompt helped me to reflect mindfully and get to know myself a little bit better.

I continued to paint too. Writing, painting, and drawing in my sketchbook offered creative outlets for my thoughts and feelings through new lenses. It didn't feel so scary as speaking my truth did and helped me realize that through the expressive arts therapeutic release was possible. Slowly, as days turned to weeks, I learned about the inner workings of my mind and body, and I invited highly skilled, intuitive therapists to journey alongside me with a measure of trust. I registered for additional courses offered through BC's Brain Wellness Program to complement medical treatments for restored brain health.

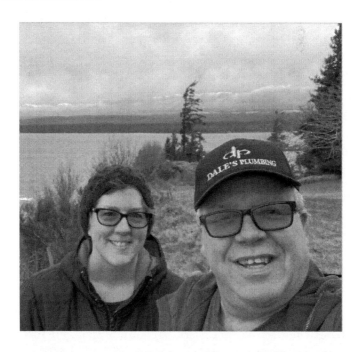

Dale and I on Nob Hill, overlooking the Strait of Georgia and Goose Spit, Vancouver Island. This was earlier that January 2021 day when I had two seizures, including the one in the crafts shop.

When I sat to journal in 2020, I typed on my laptop. I'd learned to type in high school, back in 1978, when handheld electronic communication only happened on *Star Trek*, long before personal computers or smart phones. I had a teacher with an unorthodox teaching style, who gave us each a chunk of gray waterproof tape, because duct tape fixes everything. He'd told us to cut the tape into small squares and required us to cover all the keys on the old manual typewriters that first day of class. It worked. I can type over sixty words per minute and don't need to look at the keyboard. In 2020, this skill came in handy.

Details flew from a busy brain as my fingers recorded traumatic incidents much more quickly than I could express myself. Seeing the difficult times on the page gave me the time to process and grieve losses and pain. When my brain struggled with mixed messages, my internal timekeeper set the tempo to *presto*, then raced to over 180 clicks per minute. At this frantic tempo I recorded resentment and terror, before skipping back to *allegro* intermittingly to write about running with Ollie in the North-East woods. Words flowed more easily from a lyrical soul as if dictated by a metronome clicking out a steady heartbeat.

Anytime a ride to the forest for the possibility of a walk in the woods was offered, my response was enthusiastic.

"*Yes, please,*" and my heart would skip a beat. When I was anxious my heart rate would soar like the metronome setting the tempo for a whirlwind orchestration. Except when it didn't, and I'd felt defeated making it difficult to get up off the recliner. There were too many days throughout October and November when I was thoroughly drained by cognitive loss, ripping headaches, and discouragement.

Through each day, there were so many different rhythms, and musically my brain's software glitched. My energy level soared when sunlight streamed through the canopy of the evergreen boughs. It was uplifted by the testimonial of songbirds serenading passersby. When God's creatures set the tempo, my body sang sweet contemplative prayers, and I experienced a glittery sheen of calm.

During those rare and peaceful moments in the forest and first stages of sleep each night, when my mind and body slowed, I felt drowsy and relaxed. I longed to hear exquisite collaborations by piano and cello or a songbird's rendition of Brahams' "Lullaby." I needed to be lulled and soothed by an archetypal lullaby or parent singing gently to their beloved child being rocked to sleep. Bedtime with our children was a magical time. I tried to give them everything I'd wanted. We'd cuddled, read, sang and I held them with their hearts close to mine. I missed that.

Instead, as each day ended, I prayed to my Heavenly Father. *Maranatha, Come Lord Jesus.* I was prayerful for a sleep free of nightmares and rude interruptions of up-tempo dreams about the Devil's attempt to gain a middle-aged soul in Georgia. Mine.

I asked that He might weave a new emboldened lyric into my bones and create something courageous in me. Some prayers had wings with immediate answers. Others, when I struggled to breath, had fierce headaches, and was filled with self-pity, didn't get off the ground. I didn't trust that God was listening. In those last months of the early pandemic in 2020, I struggled as many others did, just due to differing circumstances. With compromised physical, mental, and spiritual health I questioned. Were the words that flowed onto the page and images painted in my sketchbook mine? Or had they been inspired answers to prayers which fell on a deaf mute and blinded soul?

I struggled.

Insinuations by medical professionals and looks of disbelief, pity and judgement were extremely difficult to release. Those medical practitioners who'd inferred that I'd lied were difficult to forgive. Anger injured and resentment flowed from my subconscious as it travelled from my core to articulate extremities. I was reminded of my mama's voice, "If you can't say anything nice...."

Without audible expressions of grief and anger, my body battled and fought back. In error, I controlled and denied my emotions in protest. Being without self-determination was scary.

So, I controlled what I could.

~

October brought cooler temperatures and strong winds. Dale's hand found my shoulder and rested there. Its warmth radiated and reassured. I felt safe as his workworn and callused fingers moved lazily up and down my arm, releasing tension I held there. My mind was temporarily soothed as I focused on the warmth of his fingertips. Up and down, skin thirsty for touch. With his heart in his gentle hand, he left mine full.

Dale had become my full-time care partner after Mom moved out mid-September—this in addition to tirelessly working long hours alongside his business partner at Dale's Plumbing. Thankfully, they shared family-oriented priorities and by mutual agreement Dale was able to come home as needed or take time off and accompany me to most medical appointments. As time passed, this became increasingly more important, since I couldn't report back what doctors said afterwards. I didn't remember what my brain hadn't coded.

Dale had taken on the grocery shopping months earlier to prevent my exposure to COVID's Delta variant, and by October prepared most of our meals. I simply wasn't up to it.

My beloved's generosity indulged without tallying expenses. With bigheartedness he knocked off meal after meal and plated symphonies of flavour to lift my spirits. Although I felt inexpressible gratitude for his efforts, my takeaway was shame. With an inability to care for myself, read or concentrate adequately, I was now overwhelmed by bursts of electrical activity which coursed through my body unexpectedly. In a fog, I observed and witnessed a life in decline. Mine.

Heaviness settled in and took hold as I witnessed Dale's exhaustion. He shouldered most of the household responsibility and all the driving. I was ashamed to be dependent and no longer an equally contributing partner in our marriage. I was drained by the impression and realization that I now heavily taxed the finite emotional and physical resources of family and friends. Especially, Dale's. Would he be resentful in the aftermath or give up on me?

I got underway with cognitive behavioural therapy (CBT) with the aid of a web-based platform and therapist which we paid for privately. I knew I needed something. Dale repetitively said, "Whatever it takes; don't worry about the funds."

I viewed video tutorials and practiced psychoeducation techniques, which focused on aspirations, values, and strengths; monitored my mood and behaviour; tried behavioural experiments; and used a mindfulness app to regulate my breathing. I practiced making my exhale's seven seconds and longer than my four-second inhales. With a count of two I held my breath at the top and bottom of each cycle. I breathed with obsessive awareness in my attempt to get it right, as even the act of breathing was no longer instinctual.

With an editable template I endlessly typed thought-records to recognize distorted thoughts when I catastrophized. When I was absorbed in self-pity's tunnel vision, I was reminded to record what I'd been thinking just before I experienced a seizure or couldn't remember what day of the week it was. "What if?" questions grew exponentially in a mind freed from purposeful employment and unable to even complete typical day to day activities: *What if I stop breathing? What if I lost control and experienced another seizure? What if I needed a caregiver for the rest of my life?* I was only fifty-six.

Thoughts like these left me deeply discouraged and saddened. What had happened to the astute, career-minded, educational leader? What was happening to me?

~

I'd felt drawn to participate in a fundraiser for an organization called YANA (You Are Not Alone), offering support to families who need to travel for medical treatment to improve access to healthcare. It gave me a sense of purpose at a time when I felt completely isolated and dependent on others. Keith and his girlfriend, Emily, volunteered to join me and we became a cycling team aptly named The Brain Farts —an accurate reflection of my mind's state, not theirs. Our team's name had seemed a perfect descriptor of my brain's new normal. I hadn't understood why, but for some unexplained reason my brain was becoming increasingly messed up.

For the first time ever, the YANA ride would be a virtual ride. Their catchphrase had morphed during the pandemic to become: Bikes will keep us together, even when we're apart. A switch necessitated by YANA pandemic organizers who'd scrambled to shift gears when a gathering of seven hundred cyclists coming together to complete either a 50 or 100km course, wasn't permitted.

As we cycled with our freshly printed cycling bibs and plastic race numbers affixed to our bicycles I'd been feeling great. Right up until I wasn't. Without warning I lost sight of the traffic a few feet to my left, although I still felt the rush of wind with each passing car. I couldn't see Emily, who was a short distance ahead or the ditch and high tide mark to my right. In an instant my peripheral vision vanished, leaving behind a dense fog which obscured everything except where my bicycles wheels touched the ground and the pavement a short distance ahead of my front tire.

Gripped by fear, I was terrified that I'd accidentally swerve into traffic and be struck by a distracted driver if I blacked out. Seeing only the ground directly beneath my own wheels, I pedalled faster, thinking if I could just see Emily's rear tire and follow her, I might make it home. A literal brain fart occurred, and I couldn't make the safer choice to stop pedalling, slow down, and stop.

I imagined the inevitable paralysis if I crashed in vivid

detail. Somehow, I stayed hyper focused and energized by pure adrenaline until we safely reached home and stored our bikes in the back yard. Initially, I thought it best not to tell Emily, knowing she'd tell Keith, and Keith would in turn tell Dale, and I'd be restricted from one of the last remaining activities I could do independently.

Getting out on my e-bike mattered. I'd already been stripped of my independence and sanity, and I wasn't certain I could take much more loss. Dale fearing for my safety would insist that I stop cycling. He'd be right. I knew it made sense, but also knew I couldn't let him find out.

It was all too much: a body and mind in decline, the loss of my career, my driver's licence, my mom to dementia, and the realization that my future hopes and dreams may not happen ever. I might not live the long healthy life Dale had been telling me for thirty-five years I needed to prepare for. Or the twenty years without him, since women in my family appeared to live long healthy lives and Bystrom men died in their sixties.

I couldn't even begin to grasp that my brain wasn't coding information for up to eight-second intervals, that I might have blacked out causing an automobile accident or harm to others. My lack of judgment and concentration impaired my ability to read, drive, sustain attention, and remember people's names. Experiencing partial blindness and lacking sound judgement, I fully decided not to tell Emily.

Until we got home, shock set in, and I confessed my terror. And as any sane person would, she'd told Keith, who'd told Dale; just as I'd suspected.

Adding to my chagrin, Dale, after reading the epilepsy brochure at Vancouver General's epilepsy clinic waiting room, suggested, "I don't think you should have baths anymore. If you have a seizure when no one's home and lose consciousness, you could drown."

Again, another decision which made sense, but wasn't easy to accept. And swimming was out of the question, though I loved swimming. What if I ended up needing a care-aide to bathe me like Mom, but not in my eighties? Could it happen while I was still only in my fifties?

I tried to identify what I'd been thinking just before fear gripped me and I experienced central apnea or seizures but couldn't remember details. The counsellor asked, "What was the worst that could happen?" I could imagine so many possibilities, but the worst: blacking out, my lungs not filling with air, and death. I didn't want to die, so I'd been gripped by terror.

"Just because you think it, doesn't mean it's true," she'd said, as she attempted to reassure me. The counsellor tried to help me identify fears and worries and distinguish what she called my "hot thoughts"—those thoughts that seemed to be most connected to or ring the truest with what I'd experienced. For example, when I'd thought: *I'm not going to get any better and just need to accept the fact that this is my life, that my colleagues don't care about me and that's why they hadn't been in touch, and it is my fault that I lost my career in gifted education.* My anxiety and fear were invigorated by worries and I typically thought that bad things would continue to happen, that I'd be unable to cope, and be left unloved and alone.

Despite knowing that worry wouldn't really help me and, in fact, makes you focus on negativity rather than gratitude, it became increasingly more difficult to see the good.

In my online CBT lessons I learned about cognitive distortions. Magical thinking that tricked me into believing things that just weren't true. Like when Dale had come home late from work, and I'd assumed things had turned out badly without any evidence. *Was he with someone else? Had there been an accident? Had he left me?* I assumed in error that my negative thoughts accurately reflected the way things really were. If I felt lonely it must be true, that I was unlovable.

I rehearsed new patterns and ways of expressing myself after completing the CBT therapy online course and practiced conversations in my head repetitively. Then, I waited for the just right moment and blurted premeditatedly. It wasn't easy on Dale, who at times had just walked through the door, home from work. He'd be tired, frustrated, and at times hungry after an intense day. He needed to sit, unwind, and let go of stressors at work. But without thinking of consequences or his feelings, cleverly crafted words tumbled out, followed by awkward silences. Clumsy lulls, that I filled with verbal diarrhea, unable to sit in the discomfort of silence as I imagined his angry responses. Unjustified fears because, despite Dale arriving home physically and emotionally exhausted, nine times out of ten he hadn't replied in anger. He'd take his time, compose his thoughts, and respond with kindness, even when my words like weapons wounded him. He seemed to be well versed in my mama's motto, "if you can't say anything nice, don't say anything at all." Except that I needed to talk to him about all the chaos and I didn't know how.

An internal pendulum swayed back and forth, believing either that I was completely unworthy of his love and generosity or full of incredible gratitude for this beautiful human and compassionate man I'd married.

Expressing myself provoked fear and made me jittery. Fear that wasn't about Dale, his words or actions or anything he'd done. I cried when I wasn't brave enough to say anything at all and wanted to. If I cared for myself the way I cared for others I would have been able to speak up and assert myself and prioritize my needs. I was a coward.

I'd educated our children and taught students to speak up and express themselves but couldn't seem to practice what I'd preached. Momentum towards personal resilience even with counselling seemed painfully protracted. I beat myself up for the numerous perceived flaws and inadequacies I believed were true. My internal résumé was padded, and I was an imposter. I tried to believe I was secure and enough and failed.

I was never enough, and I strove not for perfection, but to be considered worthy. I had a strong innate desire to be connected, valued, and to be characterized as an effective communicator, valued human and desirable.

If I was, I wouldn't be constantly on the move—between schools, jobs, friendships, and communities. I braced for the next disconnect. If I was enough, I believed, none of this would have happened. *Was this all my fault?*

Counsellors suggested I attempt to get in touch with my feelings. Each emotion served a purpose for whole-body wellness. What good was fear? Fear kick-started me with a new desire; I wanted to look after myself and be well, if only at a snail's pace.

~

Days later, I journaled. *Some drink till they're oblivious when they're sad, angry, or filled with emotion... I stood in the shower today and cried.* I'd wanted to drive to the forest and couldn't. Hot, wet tears flowed down my cheeks. I needed my place of calm; I needed to soothe my soul and find my joy in the Northeast Woods. I'm legalistic and understood *why* I shouldn't drive. Then devilishly thought, *I might go anyway. There was no one guarding my escape, or the keys. There'd be no witnesses. No one would know but me. I could.*

Common sense prevailed. *I'm a good girl, so I don't.* I'd known that a seven-second epileptic-like discharge was long enough to cause an automobile accident, and there'd been a recent occasion on my bicycle when I hadn't coded a red light. Fortunately, I wasn't struck by a car. Unfortunately, I was frustrated by imposed limits and knowledge that robbed me of independence without an explanation or formal diagnosis. I needed my world and body to make sense.

Seven seconds. Not long enough for an epilepsy diagnosis requiring repetitive ten-second seizures, but long enough to take away almost everything I valued.

~

All was calm behind the windshield as I breathed peacefully seated beside my dear friend Rosanne. I appreciated the offered rescue from solitary confinement. Piercing winds pressed against the glass that day and rocked the vehicle as gulls swooped and glided aloft on flawless currents perfect for soaring. Waves crested and reached, then crashed atop the foamy shoreline outside Rosanne's car. In a single word, the view was magnificent.

We'd picked up lunch to go, and in comfort and safety ate as we shared stories and listened to the whipping winds and each other. My lunch, melted cheese curds layered between French fries and brown gravy—poutine—was incredibly high in total fat but totally worth the calories.

My delight on that windswept stormy afternoon allowed shoulders to fall and a long-held sigh to escape. As we sat, I'd momentarily wished I was alone and had my sketchbook to capture the magic and make it last.

~

Days passed slowly. And then on October 11 I wondered what was going on in my hands and fingers. I experienced tingling and numbness in both thumbs as well as in my index finger of my right hand. Just when I needed hand-eye coordination the most, my dexterity seemed taken. Nimbleness I took for granted vanished periodically. Opposable digits could no longer grasp tools, complete tasks, or hold a cell phone. Loss of sensation and rigidity in my hands and fingers during intimacy left me filled with shame. Fingers curled like a raptor's talons were unexpectedly flash frozen as if holding the handlebars of my e-bike. Without sensation in my fingers, a tickle went without a skilful scratch. I couldn't write, type, pick up a pencil, tool, or fork on occasion.

I perseverated under stress and questioned, *Why*? Was the new rigidity neurological, psychogenic (having a psychological cause rather than a physical one), or related to the carpel tunnel surgeries, right and left, I'd had in 2007? I was an octopus without tentacles when rigidity occurred and at a loss. I needed pointers and pinkies for zipping and buttoning and most importantly my index finger for sensory and expressive purposes like pointing and light touch discrimination. During intimacy, I imagined Dale believed I was disinterested, as I lay with clawed hands and rigid fingers, and without an ability to retract talons, or respond without shame. Why? Why was this happening to me?

I hoped against all contrary evidence that this rigidity and the increased incidence of seizures were only nightmares from which I'd wake. I didn't have a crystal ball, the clarity of a diagnosis, or medical practitioners answering my questions. Meanwhile, dexterity came and went like a silent thief in the night.

Several weeks later I travelled to Vancouver for another EEG. The procedure had just begun when I felt as if a bolt of lightning struck my skull. Current branched, sprinting from my amygdala down my whole right side: through my chest, groin, thigh, knee, calf and into my foot. The pain extended literally to the tips of each toe of my right foot.

Simultaneously, current streaked across my chest and down my left arm through a complex circuitry of nerves to my left hand and fingers. I struggled in a failed attempt to communicate what was happening to the technician. I realized, with horror when I tried to speak, that my jaw was clenched and immobilized.

"Try to relax," the technician said.

*That was good*, I'd thought. Surely the technician had noticed my brain signalling its distress in the zigs and zags being recorded in front of him. I was relieved when the pain and electrical sensations dissipated that someone other than me had finally witnessed this sort of weird event, which I'd experienced several times. I was reassured by this knowledge and audience. Certainly, the technician would alert the doctor, mark the incident by pressing the red button, as I'd been told to do during ambulatory EEGs to flag and mark an unexpected or abrupt event. Someone would observe this newly recorded data, see the epileptiform-appearing spikes and discharges, and the neurology team might finally be able to provide me with answers.

Dr. Percy would be able to explain once and for all why I repeatedly experienced nerve distress, unexplainable physical sensations, and seizure-like spells. I relaxed on the hospital gurney, closed my eyes, and allowed a small smile to take shape briefly. I'd finally be believed.

It wasn't all in my head. My brain's activity and the strange electrical impulses had been recorded for posterity. My story at last would be told.

I opened my eyes moments and looked over to where the EEG technician remained seated. I'd expected someone might rush in after they'd witnessed this traumatic incident and reassure me. It didn't happen.

"What just happened?" I asked the technician, then waited for it to be explained. This terrifying event that had rocked my body with ample physical evidence.

"Nothing out of the ordinary was recorded." Again, he encouraged me to relax.

*NOTHING!* My brain hadn't recorded or coded the event or the nth degree of trauma only I had witnessed. I was dumbstruck. It was unbelievable to hear from the technician that there was no evidence of what had just occurred.

My hands and fingers continued to register my emotional unavailability to myself and spoke volumes. *What was my body desperately trying to communicate?*

~

My body signalled that it would now be my brain's mouthpiece. It continued to advocate with fierce determination a conversation initiated seven years earlier.

With impressive resilience my body rallied and would not be denied. Initially, it had waited passively to be noticed and heard through my childhood, twenties, thirties, and forties. But by mid-October 2020, its volume intensified and left no doubts. In teacher speak, my body used its "outside voice," and like a schoolchild, cried out across the playground for an adult.

*Come and see, now!*

I heard the cry but didn't know how to acquire the care I required. I hadn't yet learned or acknowledged that my body needed health care above and below the neck. Evidence collected to date suggested neurological investigation was the specialist's primary focus. Without conscious deliberation about what lay beneath the surface, or the symptoms I experienced, I responded spontaneously without measured analysis from day to day. It was easy to believe then that my physical health needed to be prioritized; especially since I struggled to breathe and to stand unsupported.

I wasn't the only one searching for answers at the wrong address.

Meanwhile, my body continued its desperate attempt to speak a language medical specialists might comprehend. Apparently, an increased incidence of myoclonic jerks, severe headaches, and seizures wasn't enough, it determined. I was no longer able to advocate effectively for the care I required. My intelligent on-board diagnostic (OBD) system endeavoured to signal with flashing red lights, but unaware, I careened along the medical journey blinded by distraction. Specialists, my family, and I hypothesized about what caused apparent malfunctions and why vital components weren't operational. But medical practitioners failed to prioritize or recognize that fire-engine red signal that something was diabolically wrong.

Despite speculation and without a therapeutic approach to support my fragmented state of mind, I continued to trust the health care system without reproach. What other choice did I have?

~

The nightmare continued. We'll get back to you as soon as possible, eleven separate specialists inferred.

"We're still looking into this," each said, after they'd reviewed my medical records, observed, and assessed seemingly rare physical symptoms. My neuroimmunologist, cognitive stroke specialist, epileptologist, neuro-ophthalmologist, neuro-sleep disorder specialist and respirologist cared that I was suffering and tried to reassure me. But there'd been a disconnect between hearing reassurance and believing it.

~

Collaboratively, in 2020, it was agreed and communicated by my neuroimmunologist that I be tentatively diagnosed with autoimmune encephalitis and referred to an infusion clinic to begin treatments in the hope that a boost to my immune system would support wellness, with Rixmyo. A drug also administered in oncology for the treatment of non-Hodgkin's lymphoma and chronic lymphocytic leukemia. Scary? Yes.

"Perhaps there's an unknown antibody, one that we can't test for yet because it hasn't been discovered, that's causing the body's immune system to be distressed," I was told. Surprisingly this reassured me because I was desperate for a diagnosis, and it seemed the specialist wasn't willing to give up in his efforts to determine the cause of what ailed me.

Meanwhile, Dale agreed that I should privately seek out an occupational therapist to support me with strategies to complete daily tasks.

By the end of October 2020, cognitive loss made it difficult to remembers friends' and colleagues' names and what day of the week it might be. I continued to see a massage therapist for relief from stress and chronic low back pain. I carried on with cognitive behavioural therapy online, which I paid for privately in addition to various counsellors, while I waited for a phone call and intake from a psychiatric nurse in the Comox Valley.

Yes, health care is provided in Canada, but not always easily accessible. There are people who travel to the US and other countries for medical treatment and surgeries rather than wait. I wondered how many Canadians die while they wait for care or required surgeries, which only elevated an already anxious mind.

Waiting was more than discouraging, it was beyond hard. It overwhelmed an already taxed mind and body. I missed my life. I yearned to drive, work, and enjoy lunches with colleagues. I longed to be socially active and teach again. Travel during a pandemic wasn't an option, or in our budget. I needed to be patient. I didn't want to be a patient.

~

In 2013, it had been my mother who waited for a ride, after I'd discouraged her from driving at night. In 2020, it was my turn. My GP recommended that I apply for access to Handy-Dart transportation services, and I was assessed by an occupational therapist. Now, I was the one standing, waiting, peering out the plate-glass living room window as I waited for the Handy-Dart bus to take me shopping. I needed to get out, more than I'd needed to shop.

I paced back and forth killing time. Without the energy to get around independently on foot, or to use public transit, I now needed mobility services to regain independence, especially if I wanted to get to the mall. I bided time and listened for the ping and reminder on my watch as I flitted about, and up and down the stairs in our split-level home, tidying up, and adding load after load to the washer and drier. At times, I couldn't sit still.

I'd exhausted myself in the process and later had to sit on the sidewalk and lean against a cold brick wall outside the shopping center. I struggled for breath, not because of wearing a mask, but because I didn't know when the Handy-Dart might return. I felt like I might pass out, as I waited for the driver's arrival for the return trip home, which made me uneasy. Chairs everywhere it seemed had been removed or were considered an inconvenience to those who had to wipe and sanitize them. Public restrooms previously available for customers were closed. Both contributed to my discomfort and inconvenience as I sat exhausted and overwhelmed, struggling to breathe.

"Do you need a hand?" the driver asked after stopping to pick me up and opening the doors.

"Yes, please."

"You should have called," he said. "I could have come

back earlier."

I was grateful for rides, although offers by friends to get out and about were offered less and less as pandemic-related fear escalated. The BC's Health Minister recommended that we "not hug outside our safe six." Safe six, meaning a group of six friends or extended family members that was consistent for everyone involved.

Dale and I worked diligently to limit our interactions to the recommended guidelines. Shopping just wasn't the same with someone loitering close by as I browsed, to ensure my safety should I have an event. I imagined they stood impatiently and wondered how long it might take for me to hurry up and finish so they could get home after they'd offered to give me a lift.

On the morning of October 9, I hovered and paced, knowing the psychiatric nurse from community health was scheduled to call at 10:00 a.m. What would she ask? Would she believe me, and understand the embarrassment I felt at needing a psychiatrist? The doctor's referral back in March had suggested I suffered from anxiety and depression. It wasn't that, I told myself. I just needed the doctors to know what was wrong with me and how difficult it had been to have experienced scary side effects from the various experimental drug trials I'd been prescribed that didn't seem to help.

It felt like a decade but had only been ten months since I was able to drive myself to work. With ease and few burdens, I'd joyfully welcomed colleagues and students to the Library Learning Commons, as a teacher-librarian. I was thrilled to be closing in on the completion of my teacher-librarian certification through Queen's University and facilitated learning for active young minds. Teaching fed my insatiable desire to learn and fueled my intellectual curiosity. I'd arrive home satisfied that I was inspiring students and completing meaningful work. I'd happily change into my running gear energized by joy. I'd return home tired and sweaty but glowing and spirit-filled. I'd have enough residual energy to prepare homemade macaroni and cheese, a fresh green salad, and cheerfully welcome Dale. That was then.

Now I sat with a cup of tea, my thoughts like rising bubbles.

There was still another twenty-nine minutes till the psychiatric nurse was scheduled to call.

Was I discouraged? I was. Why did it take so long to get answers when there seemed abundant physical evidence that my body wasn't functioning as it should? I was frightened when I awoke exhausted, and my chest wasn't rising or filling with air. Instead, I was filled with terror when my brain seemed to forget to signal my lungs to breathe. Why were my hands constantly numb and lacking sensation?

Recent brain scans continued to report seven-second long epileptiform-appearing spikes and discharges, but nothing more. It was easy to cease believing specialists would discover what I needed most: answers.

Minds worldwide were laser-focused as we collectively held our breath and waited for life-saving vaccines. I was a single seven-second blip on an EEG readout.

I tried to remain hopeful and optimistic, but it was tough to persevere seven years later. Was Job told while he waited for God to answer his prayers, "Your symptoms are psychogenic?" Had they also inferred that the horrible skin sores Job suffered were all in his head?

Even Job got disheartened as he waited and said, "God has discouraged me. The Almighty has filled me with terror." (Job 23:16)

I wasn't surprised to be routinely asked, "Have you thought of harming yourself?" This followed up with, "Have you considered suicide or made a plan?"

*I hadn't.* Although, it occurred to me that had I not been an articulate, capable individual with strong support systems and a tight-knit family, *I might have.*

Every day I struggled. I continued to attempt advocacy and became more and more discouraged after my efforts didn't seem to hasten the process or slow the physical decline. What was it that had taken a firm hold on me?

Knowing I might stop breathing at any time not because I was suicidal, but because it had happened once briefly and might again, caused anxious thoughts.

Like Job, I was terrified.

~

After the forty-five-minute-long appointment with the psychiatric nurse, she'd summed up our conversation by saying, "I understand that you're anxious and depressed." *No shit, Sherlock.* You'd be anxious and depressed, too, if you'd been waiting six plus years for answers.

The psychiatric nurse, concluding the appointment, said, "Jocelyn, you're not super connected to your emotions." She hadn't listened with curiosity or apparently heard me at all.

I was told I'd hear from the psychiatrist by the end of November. *End of November? That was another seven weeks away.*

*I'm a volcano on fire, ready to erupt.* Surely, she hadn't thought she'd be able to understand me after a brief telephone call.

"Not super connected." *Brains like mine think with heightened, intense feelings and a full spectrum of emotions.*

I journaled October 19 about the prior few weeks:

```
"They took my brain away," Mom told me
last week. They? Who's they? I'd wondered.
Apparently, they've come for mine too. But my
mind and body are fighting back.
     That day, my mind was the victor. But
victory celebrations don't last. There's always
```

another battle.

Yesterday, I experienced anger, fear, sadness, confusion, joy, and concern for a friend's well being—all in a single day. Since ringing in the New Year, January 1, 2020, I've continued to experience life in vivid pictures with big, intense emotions. My body is hyperaware. Perhaps the psychiatric nurse had assessed, but not questioned, what I hadn't said. I'd been hyper aroused, and literally and figuratively armoured for self protection.

She hadn't asked about the traumatic incident at Vancouver General when bolts of pain, like lightning, struck. Bolts that split and fractured, like blood pumped through arteries to extremities.

She sat, I imagined, at a remote home office, with her cell phone in hand and a prerequisite list of intake assessment questions. This, while I sat easily distracted and with impaired cognition. I'd tried to provide answers, but a mind fueled by fear subconsciously withheld its tale.

I'd listened to the psychiatric nurse, heard her questions, and attempted to respond in an intelligent manner, but was distracted by an ambulance racing through my neighborhood and was triggered.

Who might be strapped to the gurney and being raced to the ER? I imagined the victim's loved ones and bodily experienced their angst. Too easily, I imagined myself experiencing their shock after learning a loved one had been in a horrific accident. I know the pain of grief without a road map to help heal hurt.

What might have caused the collision and

the caller to dial 911, I'd pondered? I recreated the imagined scene and aftermath in precise detail. The ambulance attendants, the traffic slowing, drivers with furrowed brows pressed to glass staring, and the mangled car seat still buckled into the broken wreck. With magical thinking, I easily envisioned the parent and driver, now laying silent in a recently zipped body bag.

Was it an infant, someone's beloved child, and the only surviving family member now being rushed to the emergency room? Where were my loved ones at that exact moment, I'd worried. Was it possible that a family member or friend lay strapped to the stretcher inside the wailing ambulance? I hadn't imagined the sirens.

I'd answered the psychiatric nurse's questions to the best of my ability and afterward escaped, either literally or figuratively, to my place of calm.

I transported myself back to where and when I'd last caressed droplets of dew. Drops which dangled after the cool of night, as I wandered my favourite and familiar paths in the Northeast Woods. I know them well.

When I tread gently through the forest's early morning mist, I'm alone but never lonely. God finds and meets me there. I wipe away the spider's silk that embraces my face and wraps my skin in a cocoon of lacework. Brushing it from my skin my heart's tempo slows, as it needed to.

I'm connected to my emotions; I just can't verbalize the depth and magnitude of loss and grief my mind and body have endured.

Don't say, "I understand."

~

I was at a crossroad and ill-prepared for an unwelcomed guest on October 19, when a furry rodent checked in for a long stay. I presumed he'd crept in seeking warmth and comfort, between sunset and first light. I imagined he sensed the warmer temperature within as he darted along his nightly foraging route. Not wanting to fall prey to either an owl or something slithering, he'd trusted his acute hearing and stopped briefly to investigate. Perhaps he'd been nervous and panicked, running inside to escape threat.

~

*What's this?* I wondered as I knelt for closer inspection thinking it must be a crumb or fallen kitchen scrap. In horror, I thought it appeared to be mouse feces. It couldn't be, I told myself, and then hadn't thought too much about it until later when I headed downstairs to the basement and noticed the still opened sliding glass door. Later I learned the feces were those of a very savvy rat.

How could I have been so stupid?

Easily, my brain wasn't working properly. The day before I'd gone out the sliding patio door, thinking, *I'll be right back*. Then I'd headed upstairs to the deck via the outside staircase and returned into the house through the French doors on the upper level. The opened lower door, forgotten.

He needed to be eliminated.

Already in an elevated state with my first steroid infusion of Rixymo only weeks away, obsessive behaviours kicked in. I'd vacuumed, wiped down every surface, and thrown out anything that bore evidence of the rat's trespasses against us. With robust energy I hadn't known I was still capable of I was driven as if an expectant soon to be new mother in her thirty-ninth week. She'd have been on a mission to nest, while my mission was to find and destroy one. Dale called the exterminator and set a trap line.

I needed to hear "SNAP" and see his whiskered deceased

body.

~

My family believed I was an assertive human all along. It simply wasn't true. When acquiring care and advocating for others, yes, but not for myself. Hadn't they witnessed my transformation to silence and changed body language? I hadn't been speaking up about my concerns. I believed erroneously that my thoughts communicated my anxiety and that others could read my fear. I wasn't aware I sounded assertive or that appearances could be so deceptive. November left me completely out of sync with my body and emotions.

At the recommendation of a close friend, who'd started a therapeutic relationship with a counsellor she trusted, she suggested that I perhaps give her counsellor a call. Why I waited so long to follow through and seek mental health support could only have been a result of critical self-judgement. Self-stigma impacted how I thought about myself and my relationships with others and thus affected my initial motivation to recover.

Various incidents without prerequisite distress tolerance skills made me believe I didn't deserve what I needed. I'd modified my social expectations and then adopted negative feelings about myself. After being told I was unprofessional and labelled a liar I'd accepted my thoughts as truth, and it led to disempowerment and a decreased quality of life. I subsequently experienced both physical and cognitive decline

I robbed myself of self-esteem and self-control without realizing it and was in a constant state of hypervigilance. Seven years of complex physical health challenges had taken a toll leaving me helpless and broken. I needed support to help break my silence, get out of my head, and connect with my heart. I wanted to believe Dale when he'd tell me, "You're beautiful." But I didn't.

~

In the chaos of everything that happened I felt spiritually lost and struggled to pray. Without a daily habit of prayer my journal became a tool for lament. There I expressed what I was unable to speak aloud. Writing became my heart's song and the beginnings of a wisdom tale of humility. What began as therapeutic became nourishment and helped support healing. I'd needed healing as my mind and body shut down.

Much later I would weave documented journal threads recorded through 2020 into storytelling fabric and a tale with a surprise ending. As I wielded my pen it allowed my body to have its say, and for my heart to listen with curiosity. I had head knowledge about co-regulation, and social emotional intelligence much earlier. I'd taught my students and our children to have teachable spirits and to advocate for themselves. Head knowledge just hadn't found its way to my heart.

*Lord, help me sing a new song of unconditional love and self-acceptance. I need a brave heart, courage to trust, and the Holy Spirit to breathe gratitude and love into each note and verse.*

*Amen.*

~

I didn't have the courage and hadn't found the stage, the audience, or the individual I could trust, yet.

Some incidents needed to be planted and discovered, discharged, and liberated. Others needed to become irrelevant and allowed to scatter into the wind.

Finally, I would see a psychiatrist.

# CHAPTER SEVENTEEN

### Flight, Fright or Fail

"Are you okay?" family and friends would ask. They couldn't read my body's language or hear through the invisible shield I unknowingly held. My innate survival instincts persisted, thankfully, while my body had given up altogether.

I'd believed myself safe and been proven wrong time and time again. By employers, by insurance companies selling security, and by my own body. I didn't dare speak truth to gain power. I tried to explain again and again that I needed help. Why couldn't anyone solve the difficult puzzle that was me? How might I learn the deeper telling truths?

I imagined embryonic wings and used my limited strength to hatch. I needed help, lacked trust, and had lost faith. I had difficult choices to make and was perplexed by the unsolved riddle of seizures, headaches, and cognitive loss. Deciding what to do was tough. Without a fully functioning prefrontal cortex I pecked and stabbed to perforate the semipermeable membrane and break through the discomfort. My heart wanted to fly, but my soul had plummeted and dissolved into tears.

It was November and I prepared for infusions of a

biologic called Rixmyo. Prescribed collaboratively by my team of neurologists to keep at bay an unknown antibody. An antibody which might be warring with my immune system and causing seizures.

I travelled November 4 and 18, in a van provided by the non-profit Wheels for Wellness Society, to and from non-emergency medical appointments. Dale was needed at work, so I'd offered to travel alone.

"I'll be fine." I said, to reassure myself as much as for Dale.

Wheels for Wellness Society needed to significantly adjust their operations at the height of the pandemic. They'd added Plexiglass and plasticised barriers between seats and only transported a maximum of three passengers to protect both volunteer drivers and clients.

*Here we go*, I thought, stepping into my Saran Wrapped transport cubicle the morning of November 4. Despite reading the prerequisite information about the drug trial and what to expect, I packed more than I needed for what I'd been told could be a 6–7-hour infusion. My mind raced, trying to make sense of its flood of neurotic questions. A pharmaceutical rep had called prior to ensure I was indeed who I said I was, and confirm that I met the fundamental parameters of their research study.

"You do have an MS diagnosis?" she asked.

*Multiple sclerosis?*

"No, not that I'm aware of," I'd responded, and she ended the call without further questions or confirmation that I'd be eligible for the trial just two days away. All she said was that she'd check into my eligibility and let me know.

"Is this Jocelyn I'm speaking to?" the same rep started with on her follow-up call. "You do in fact meet the prerequisite eligibility requirements." Then without further clarification she confirmed that I needed to be at the clinic where they'd send the medication the following day. My first series of infusions had been scheduled two weeks apart. I would return to the clinic for a second series in March 2021. *Wait, did I have MS?* The call hadn't created calm or been reassuring. Her call hadn't really been about me, or about steadying the whitecaps which threatened even before the storm. I waited for the hours to pass, the morning to come, and for the duration of the hour-long drive south from the Comox Valley to Nanaimo. Once there, I tried to read and signed numerous releases I didn't really understand as the IV technician searched for the "just right" vein.

"You're a hard target," I'd been told on more than one occasion.

Riximyo, a biopharmaceutical drug designed to have active properties like Rituximab, an expensive name brand drug, might be capable of recognizing the yet undiscovered antigen, which caused my body distress. Riximyo, my neuroimmunologist and neurology team hoped, would slow and eliminate the increasingly intense seizures. I wasn't certain it would work, but anything at this stage was worth a try. Could my health get any worse? *It probably would.*

I'd said yes to the experimental drug treatment and signed on the dotted line.

Another risk factor, just in case I hadn't been overwhelmed enough, I was told *after* those first infusions. The predicted success rate of new COVID-19 vaccines, which Americans and Canadians expected to be rolled out mid-December, were expected to have 50 percent reduced effectiveness for immunocompromised individuals. *I* was now immunocompromised.

Between infusions I balanced visits now deemed essential for Mom, who was then settled into long-term care. Provincial restrictions had tightened since September, and visitors were no longer allowed in to visit their loved ones in all Vancouver Island Health Authority's care homes. Fortunately for me, Mom had been placed in a publicly funded community of care called Providence Living. Their vision is to completely reimagine the experience of seniors and others in need of dementia care, and they allowed both social and essential visitation throughout 2020. On the edge of sanity, this hadn't been the factor to tip the precarious balance.

Other than walking to visit Mom three times a week, I stayed home. We'd become each other's life-support line.

I put a sign on the front door stating in bold red lettering:

STOP. SOMEONE IN THIS HOUSE HAS A WEAK IMMUNE SYSTEM.

And in fine print below: *Those who are immune-compromised are more likely to contract the coronavirus (COVID-19) and experience life-threatening complications. Please leave packages/deliveries on the doorstep. If you need us, please call.*

Thinking about "life-threatening complications," and mindful of what was happening in the United States, I instituted strict protocols for who I'd open the door to: Dale, Keith, and Emily (Keith's girlfriend) were allowed. And Kristen, if at some point she was legally allowed to travel to another health region.

Simultaneously, *Forbes Magazine* reported "November 2020's Grim COVID-19 Totals" and unprecedented death tolls. There were record-shattering new infections recorded in the United States. In November alone, 37,000 deaths.

Canadians listened and were infused with statistics broadcast twenty-four seven. Canada's national death toll to date, as of November 29, 2020, had just passed 12,000. *Twelve thousand people were dead! Holy crap.*

Since the first worldwide COVID-19 infection was broadcast January 2020, there'd been a total of only 435 COVID-19 related deaths in British Columbia, and six on Vancouver Island. Every death mattered and was someone's loved one. I was all caps AFRAID.

By accessing my inherent creativity, my mind, which had gone to frightening places after each seizure, was soothed. I sought solace through November amidst a life filled with chaotic uncertainty. I slowly learned that my body and mind craved opportunities to synthesize intense events and reflect, move, pray, rest, recharge, and simply be.

Words flowed in the sacred, safe spaces as I learned to use mindfulness, and created breathing room between thoughts and poetic words and gaps between the difficulties. I'd needed periods of time to fill my senses and feel alive. Workshop facilitators from the BC Brain Wellness Program used simple guided meditations, accessible through Zoom workshops, to help participants rediscover their imaginations and creative confidence. I was able to reconstruct new support systems online through this programing at a time I was stuck in uncertainty, isolation, and immune compromise.

I was able to be present for myself there—witness my beauty and creativity, massage my spirit, and find joy. It took a conscious effort and hard work to re-establish a practice of prayer during a season when I still didn't trust my prayers would be answered.

*Holy Spirit, find me here in this bubble of solitary silence. My body is your dwelling place and I need your help, Lord, to take good care of it. Heal me, restore me, and make me whole again, so that my inner beauty might shine through the safeguards I've erected. In the spaces between my thoughts, Lord, remind me to pray. In the gaps between my difficulties, shelter me close to you. Amen.*

The morning of November 13, there'd been a short but impactful seizure during intimacy. Loving touches cease when two lovers stare down fear created by a seizure. The heart speeds and intimacy ends with panic. Will the seizure stop?

Disheartened, I swiveled and sat on the side of our bed. I opened my mouth and words came without a plan. For the first time in years, I prayed aloud for myself while Dale listened.

With elbows out and thumbs facing forward I pressed my fingers into my low back and gently arched. Eyes closed I let my prayer float upwards in the darkened bedroom as Dale held me close.

*"Jesus, help me."* A simple prayer, but it was all I had.

~

As I turned the calendar page to December, I learned that my first psychiatric appointment would be Wednesday the ninth, and added it to my Google Calendar, where I meticulously kept track of dates and appointments that I had no hope of committing to memory. I hadn't a clue about what to expect during a telephone psychiatric appointment, but the eleven months wait left me hopeful.

~

"Hello?"

"Hello. Jocelyn?"

"Yes, this is Jocelyn."

"It's Dr. Rothchild, calling from the Wellness Center, at the North Island Hospital."

The valley's new hospital, named North Island Hospital – Comox Valley Campus, opened in October 2017, and already I'd been admitted more times in 2020 than I'd been hospitalized in my lifetime.

My psychiatrist asked more questions, and I responded. The arrival of the long-awaited appointment date had arrived, and my story tumbled out. I spoke until I stopped. He listened with few interruptions. I imagined him taking copious notes. I speak quickly when I'm propelled by fear. My colleagues might say that I arrive to work earlier than most, that I'm driven, that I never miss a deadline, and that I'm always willing to help. They might tell you that I fill my schedule to ensure I'm busy. What they may not know—and I would never share—is that beneath the surface, I'm fighting a constant churn of anxiety, and afraid that I'll disappoint others. This is what drives me and why I don't find it easy to sit still.

The psychiatrist questioned and I answered. We talked about current medications I was taking, the recent Rituximab infusions neurologists had recommended for autoimmune encephalitis, and he suggested diagnoses of PTSD, OCD, and generalized anxiety.

We discussed the loss of my treasured position, as a gifted education specialist, and my inability to manage loss and grief. He recorded that I was currently taking brivaracetam, a generic of the brand name Brivlera, as well as the dosage I had previously been prescribed by my neurology team.

Brivaracetam belongs to a class of antiepileptics, commonly used, in addition to other medications, to treat and prevent seizures for people with epilepsy. It works by affecting the transmission of nerve signals in the brain. I was also on topiramate, sold under the brand name Topamax, yet another drug used to treat epilepsy and prevent migraines. Both were medications prescribed after expert consultation and much deliberation by my team of neurologists. In addition, I was taking a low dose of sertraline, an anti-anxiety medication, since coming home from my August 2020 admission at Vancouver General's neurology ward. Each medication had proven to be the best option available with the least destructive side effects.

My psychiatrist prescribed an increased dose of sertraline to treat my depression, panic attacks (anxiety), obsessive compulsive disorder (OCD), and post-traumatic stress disorder (PTSD). It made sense to me; that an increased dose could be beneficial, and I'd agreed to titrate to the higher dosage.

Sertraline had improved my mood, sleep, and energy level plus decreased my anxiety and unwanted thoughts. The notion that it would additionally lessen my recent panic attacks gave me hope. Dr. Rothchild recommended that between my next telephone appointment I complete the first several modules of *Assert Yourself!*, offered by the Government of Western Australia's Center for Clinical Interventions online. Do It Yourself (DIY) therapy was the prescribed antidote for what ailed me. I found contents of these modules helpful but wasn't confident it was what I required to see restored physical health.

I trusted, increased the dosage of sertraline as had been suggested, and completed the assertiveness training modules, then waited.

With Christmas just two weeks away, traditional celebrations with extended family and friends gathered around the dining table wasn't permitted. There were national and provincial restrictions about visiting in one another's homes. Christmas it seemed was destined to be unlike any other. And, as 2020 ended, I still hadn't been diagnosed with epilepsy, or any of the other suspected neurological conditions.

*What was wrong with me?* Why was I losing my mind? Was it any surprise I couldn't trust easily? Would I recover from whatever was taking me down?

My family later told me they'd discussed the possibility of me not making it through to the end of the year. Perhaps I wouldn't live to be fifty-seven.

Dale, medical specialists, friends, family, and God each waited patiently for me to trust. Each deserved and had earned trust, but my surrender of control wasn't imminent.

I hadn't trusted, although I said I did. I repetitively reassured Dale when he'd say, "You don't trust me!"

"But I do. I do trust you!"

He'd known the truth and was partially correct. I don't trust easily. In the depths of discouragement December 10, I wrote in my journal:

> Going out onto the limb with you. You're leading me, and I choose to follow, cautiously. Gently you nudge and offer self determination, sparks of hope, and safety. All that's required of me is surrender. But I guard my heart jealously, and it isn't easy. It won't be easy. I've counted on self control for a lifetime. And you ask, "How's that worked out for me, so

```
far?"
    I'll choose trust and follow your lead.
Keep watch over me. Will I be safe, can I trust
your words and actions? I hope so. I'm counting
on you.
```

I've protected myself with silence and observed that speaking power into my truth causes conflict. I couldn't and can't manage conflict well. So, I guard a tender heart despite the knowledge that standing-on-guard exacerbates conflict. The tension has brought me to my knees. I was at another crossroads and exhausted by an unwelcomed guest.

~

*Heavenly Father, I surrender my fears, hopes, and dreams. My all. Today, Lord, I'll wait no longer. I'm waving the white flag, surrender control, and choose trust. I long to rest in Your peace and be assured of Your mercy. I need You, Father God. As my living presence, my center, and my all in all. Help me to be still, listen and rest in your always available, unconditionally loving arms. I am your beloved child and loved. Thank you, Jesus. ~ Amen.*

This prayer, I prayed December 12. I'd known that in my own strength I wouldn't be able to overcome my fears, rid our home and sanctuary of a fiendish rat, or learn to trust. I'd needed a Heavenly Father, the Holy Spirit, and Jesus, three in one. I needed an Almighty, all-capable, unconditionally loving, merciful God.

~

Rattus rattus, nicknamed after week one and still hiding five weeks later, had a new alias The Furry Fiend. He'd caused irreparable harm. Dale unloaded hundreds of pounds of chewed and destroyed belongings at the landfill. From the back of a Dale's Plumbing Ltd. cube van, he threw damaged furniture, chewed ceiling tiles, appliance wiring, the burner control wiring harness from our gas range, our couch, various antiques which had belonged to my mom, and box after box of stored teaching resources. The sum of my career I'd tucked away, pending my return to work from the full medical leave that my neurology team recommended nearly a year before. I hadn't the heart yet to give my teaching supplies away. But fearing the uninvited guest would continue its rampage, I gifted most of my treasured professional belongings in December 2020. It seemed I might never teach again. That thought was soul-crushing.

It was heartbreaking witnessing valued belongings in ruin. The Furry Fiend had even picked away with its rodent incisors most of the wood filler between the oak panels of our dining room table. It had no concern for a table I'd purchased with my very first teaching pay cheque in 1986, and urinated and left feces everywhere.

Thoroughly disgusted, I washed and put clean linens over the table top each morning, after sanitizing what remained of the wooden surface. Exterminators set out poison the first week of December and returned periodically, pressured by my angst without noticeable success. I was told I may have to wait till the poison takes effect and that the rat may crawl into a wall to die. It could take weeks before a putrid odour told the tale of its demise.

They'd returned December 18, headed downstairs and used the ladder to open several of the chewed ceiling tiles, where there were also traps set.

"We got him!"

*Had I heard correctly?* I'd been upstairs and immediately headed down the front stairs to confirm what I thought I'd heard, before celebrating. Confirmation was a necessity.

My shoulders collapsed as exhaled breath escaped. At long last I'd be able to breathe in sweetness, like the moments after you wave goodbye to guests who've overstayed their welcome. This, as the masked and gloved pest control agent met me on the stairs. Pinched in fingers protected by thick leather gloves he'd held up the trap and trophy.

"This is one shiny coated, well-fed furry, Black Rat."

At 10:58, Friday morning, December 18, 2020, I texted

Dale, Keith and Kristen on Fam Jam our family's group chat:

"The [deceased] rat, has left the building." Except in my excitement, I'd misspelled deceased as "diseased."

At 11:17, I added, "Hallelujah!!!" It had been fifty-nine days of hell, not on earth, but in our house.

~

On Christmas Eve, my extremely thoughtful neurologist, Dr. Percy, called. She called surprisingly late on a day when most folks, I'm certain, had already headed home to celebrate and prepare for Santa's arrival. But she knew I would want to hear the results of my EEG from December 9 before she headed home from work for the holidays.

The multimodal approach, which she'd recommended collaboratively with my team of neurologists, included seizure medication, immunotherapy, counselling, and now psychiatry, in addition to the complementary brain health classes I was still enjoying through UBC's Brain Wellness Program. This approach seemed to have decreased the epileptiform spike and wave discharges from numerous half-a-second to seven-second spikes noted on previous EEG's, to discharges that were now at most three seconds long. This was exciting news and lifted our spirits.

As global citizens stood six feet apart, wore masks, and stayed home in isolation, we collectively rang in the New Year. Everyone it seemed agreed, it was time to escort out 2020 and the pandemic and return to NORMAL.

Except in the Bystrom household, January 3, the proverbial shit hit the fan.

# CHAPTER EIGHTEEN

**The Shit Hits the Fan, and I Fall**

A new season of terror swept in on January 3, 2021—a year I'd hoped would bring healing and peace. I was awakened just before 4:30 a.m. by an odd feeling. Next, as if I hadn't experienced sufficient emotional distress during the past twelve months, bolts of electricity found new neural pathways. Like thunder, the seizure struck out of the blue and disorganized electrical impulses bolted and zigzagged along the spinal cord.

The seizure was scary enough that Dale, usually calm during emergencies, awakened instantaneously. He instinctively knew this one was different. First, he grabbed his phone out of reflex to take a video, as my neurologist had requested in the event of a significant seizure, and then scrambled instead to dial 911.

It was my first full body, complex seizure and extremely different than the short but intense seizures I'd experienced during intimacy. Neither of us knew what to anticipate. My jaw without warning went rigid. Eyelids squeezed shut and lips were stuck together. I breathed with difficulty through my CPAP machine and its nasal pillow mask, designed to make sleeping more comfortable for those like me, who are naughty stomach sleepers.

Sheer force of will wasn't enough for me to reopen eyelids or my mouth. My right hand and arm lay bent and deadened while my left, which had been stretched out under my head and pillow while I'd slept, beat animatedly above the funny bone, as if it belonged to a member of an airport's ground crew guiding a jet in from the runway. Periodically, my left hand hit my head.

With new superhuman strength my body contracted then discharged energy invariably. Legs bent at the knees appeared to be glued together as they pumped in and out, stripping sheets and blankets from where they'd been tucked.

My brain, too, seemed super-charged with significant horsepower, like a gasoline engine infused with nitrous oxide. With more oxygen available during a seizure my body wholly distressed me with its monumental power and force.

When I heard the ambulance arriving, a chaotic mind experienced distorted thought. I'm an incredibly restless sleeper who gets tangled in pyjamas from constant tossing and turning, so don't wear any. There was no way for me to maintain control during a seizure or to ensure my privacy. Dale, as if a mind reader, consistently pulled the sheet up and over me as he'd waited for the seizure to stop, knowing I'd want some modicum of privacy when ambulance attendants entered.

Soon, medics entered our master bedroom, arriving at the bedside just as large rhythmic movements ended. I attempted to return to my pre-seizure normal by taking more relaxed breaths instead of deep gasping inhales, but it seemed almost impossible.

The weight of my head felt immense. My face and jaw were unyielding as I lay stripped of blankets and the ability to gesture or speak. Thankfully, I was still covered by a single, 300-thread count cotton sheet.

As Dale spoke to the paramedics intently observing me, my jaw finally softened.

I'd had little to no aura, the feeling most epileptics experience before a Grand Mal seizure. My seizures instead erupted without a loss of consciousness. Unlike an epileptic, who may experience tonic-clonic seizures and be rendered unconscious during a seizure, and which may cause brain damage or death. Mine seemed identical, but I was fully aware of every second as the seizure lapsed.

Dale's face afterward seemed aged by the length of the seizure and intensity of emotion, his and mine.

Keith offered to come to Comox and work remotely, doable during the pandemic. Kristen, too. They took turns through January, relieving Dale as my care partner. Dale could gratefully head to the office to catch up on paperwork, reassured that our adult children could be trusted to handle anything that arose. I'd been incredibly grateful that they'd both offered without being asked.

I wish I could say that things stabilized after the early morning of January 3, but it was the first of a string of seizures to come.

The second complex seizure occurred later that same day.

Saturday, January 9, brought *three* seizures.

I experienced repetitive grandiose movements each time of my head, trunk, arms, and legs. Large muscle groups became rigid and stiff or jerked, then uncontrollably changed in irregular, unexpected patterns. There were multiple ambulance rides in short order.

~

"You can head home whenever you're ready," the ER nurse told me on January 9, after removing my IV. She applied pressure over gauze where the needle had threaded into the vein and then secured surgical medical tape over the dressing. After putting on my own clothes, I pulled my hooded jacket on over the injection site they'd used to deliver medicine and fluids through a flexible tube.

Without further instruction, I exited the triage room in the ER and wove my way through the maze of corridors from the ER to where Dale waited parked outside the Emergency

Entrance. I'd texted him to say I was on my way, and he'd pulled up closer to the ER doors temporarily. By the time I got to the car in the loading zone and was seated and buckled my arm felt very wet.

While Dale drove, I investigated and found that blood had leaked out of the IV site without enough pressure exerted and now saturated my long-sleeved pullover and jacket. I was so thankful to be discharged that I didn't want to head back to the ER when Dale suggested it. Instead, I applied pressure, knowing that was what was required, and suggested we head straight home.

Home was a comforting sight after long hours at the ER. Shortly after Dale pulled into the driveway and we headed inside, I stripped off my bloody clothing. While I continued to apply pressure, I changed the gauze and resecured new gauze in place with tape from our trusty first aid kit. Blood hadn't flowed unchecked afterwards.

We had a small bite to eat, then Dale asked if I'd be willing to accompany him on an errand to deliver lumber to a friend. He didn't want me to be home alone since our adult children had moved out, and I hadn't wanted that either.

So, we headed out once again, this time in a Dale's plumbing truck, to meet up with his friend Steve. After dropping off the lumber with Steve, Dale asked if I felt up to a short walk. He had something in mind that he'd wanted to show me.

He helped me out of his truck's passenger seat and wrapped my body with his strong arm, a gesture that reassured.

I was still weak but loved the idea of being outdoors and of escape from catastrophic discouraged thoughts. Steve, a master craftsman, was building new cabinets for Dale's plumbing van at his shop, situated on a lovely seaside property and perfect spot to find calm. Ollie, our cocker spaniel, had tagged along on this outing, not wanting to be left at home either. Each time I had a seizure he'd come to me, distressed by each unexpected event. It seemed as if he wanted to protect me, but whined because he didn't know how.

Hand in hand we walked, my left hand lifted and secured in his, while his right arm circled around my back and lovingly held me secure. We walked across the property to the edge of the cliff featuring a gorgeous view. I was glad I'd worn the new toque that my brother-in-law Hugh hand knit to match the cable-knit sweater he'd gifted me for my last birthday.

The day's winds were strong enough that my unbound hair would have become wound up in a bird's nest and given me an earache to remember long after I'd returned indoors. The view was stunning. From this single vantage point, we were able to see across the expanse of Georgia Strait to the mainland, as well as Goose Spit, aptly named for its reach of sand formed by longshore movement and sediment carried out by the Puntledge River into Comox Bay Harbour.

Dale's arm held me grounded. We could see forever. Dale, my guardian protector, ensured there'd be no accidental stumbles if unexpected myoclonic jerks or a seizure started. There'd be no more photos of me standing alone, at the edge of a cliff, or anywhere, if Dale had any say in the decision.

We could see and were swept away by frothy whitecaps, which covered and sheltered us. Our senses were literally filled by this seascape, as winds blew clouds hurriedly across the sky. The most recent tide provided a west coast perfume that wakened me to promise. I could see all the way past Texada Island to Powell River and its pulp and paper mill, where that day stacks weren't pumping out effluent as they often are.

My mind flew up and glided like the planes air cadets at the base use as they train to be pilots. Up and away from worry I escaped, like a jet streaking across the sky or a seagull soaring on the sea breezes for the sheer delight of it. I wished once again I could fly.

All would be well, again, we wanted to believe. We stopped briefly to take a few selfies against the scenic backdrop, and then to watch the kite surfers roll, loop, and summersault with a firm grip on their kite's control bar, before heading back home.

"How are you doing? Are you up to one more stop?" Dale asked. I had to admit, I wasn't. Dale needed to be at work and supporting his business partner to ensure our plumbing business operated smoothly during the pandemic, and this knowledge weighed heavily on me, as Dale prioritized my care. I shouldered guilt at being so high-maintenance and needy. He hadn't prioritized his needs or the business for months.

He took the most direct route home and didn't say anything, which made me feel bad. He was fully present for me, and if distracted by anxious thoughts about work, he hadn't let on or allowed his concerns to impact my health. But I noticed. His stress level was apparent, and I worried he would have a heart attack.

The short outing had happily exhausted me, and I reclined in the living room. Dale brought me a cool glass of water and asked if I needed anything else. I requested my CPAP machine, hoping it might help re-establish a more regular rhythm when I felt breathless.

I'd no sooner settled and closed my eyes when I got that funny feeling again.

I tried to alert Dale but was temporarily mute as another seizure got underway. I attempted to snap my fingers to get his attention, like before, but this time was unable to gesture. This second seizure, in less that twelve hours, came on hard and fast and included large muscle group movements that rocked, lurched, jerked, and convulsed.

Dale came to me even without a signal and spoke my love language. His words reassured, and he kept up a constant chatter about anything that came to mind that might distract me from the seizure. We realized after previous seizures that just hearing his voice, which engaged and distracted, helped seizures conclude more quickly. I wouldn't remember the specifics of what he said, but that didn't matter. Sensing his face and gentle presence tethered me.

We talked in bits and bursts after seizures. We each processed what we'd experienced in our own unique way. We hugged a lot when words eluded us. Afterwards, we'd both been fragile. I became afraid to sit and/or recline, though had no other option as my eyelids drooped.

Dale became very quiet; he's a strong silent processor of his emotions. He hovered and was ever ready, twenty-four seven. Dale probably hadn't realized the exorbitant cost when at twenty-one he vowed to love me in sickness or in health, and replied, "I do!"

He watched me sleep. I wondered, as I lay with my eyes closed attempting sleep, if he thought, *Would this breath be her last? Might this be her last birthday, or our last year married?* He didn't dare sleep. It haunted me to think of how much worry and sleeplessness I caused. His version of the past few years, though he didn't choose to share it, must have been a nightmare of epic proportion.

In the silence, which was most of the time, I worried a lot about Dale.

Seizure #2 lasted just over thirteen minutes. Dale had called 911, for the second time. He appeared relieved, I thought, as I last saw his face before the ambulance carried me away. I wasn't his burden to shoulder anymore. I wondered if he'd been able to rest after I left, though I knew he wouldn't. When he worries, Dale's a doer. He doesn't sit still.

~

Thankfully as the ambulance arrived at the ER, another ambulance attendant recognized me from a previous 911 call he'd attended at our home. He was finishing up in nearby triage room and told the medics who wheeled me in that his daughter suffered from nonepileptic seizures. He explained that he believed this might be what was happening to me as I seized once again on the gurney.

The paramedic coached me through seizure #3, which had started in the ambulance as we arrived at the hospital, as

Dale would have, had he been present. He spoke to receiving nurses and doctors in the ER about psychogenic nonepileptic seizures (PNES) and reiterated that I probably didn't require Ativan.

*Nonepileptic seizures?* I'd wondered. *Is that what's going on with me?* As a result, doctors hadn't given Ativan, a drug which I later learned was standard protocol during an epileptic event.

While I waited in a triage room, the attending doctor left to communicate with a neurologist at Vancouver General. He returned to say that the doctor from VGH had said that my status wasn't emergent. I didn't require immediate life-saving treatment, as I had during the hot-stroke protocol in July 2020. I fell into the delayed category, as a patient who required medical intervention, but not with any urgency. The neurologist told my triage doctor that a transfer to the SIU, or Seizures Investigation Unit, wouldn't happen till at least Monday. I was released from the hospital and headed home again after the attending ER doc apologized, "I tried; however there doesn't seem much we can do." He observed my puffy eyes, and dilated pupils as I listened, and with empathy offered me an out. "If you're afraid, you can stay."

Despite my fear, I chose not to ask to be admitted. I'm a quick study and knew that without a neurology department there was no point. At least at home I'd be comfortable, have Dale, and not need to spend the night imagining the worst. I didn't want to listen to alarms beeping, or distressed roommates crying out in pain, as I had for seven nights in July 2020.

I could have a seizure at the hospital or at home and the result would be the same. The seizure would start, I would seize, and it would end. That had been my experience to date. The only variables I'd learned were the length and intensity I would be required to endure.

I chose to go home, and to Dale.

I started to believe my seizures, although extremely intense, might just be nonepileptic, although I didn't really understand what that meant. Curious minds need to research and understand what they fear, especially mine, so I took the time to learn about the various kinds of seizures and tried to conceptualize the difference between epileptic and nonepileptic. However, a brain that's experienced significant cognitive decline can't always understand or remember. I didn't need to Google seizures to know they were scary. Lived experiences had taught me that. I only needed to find reliable scholarly research and be assured that death wasn't a probable outcome or in my near future. I didn't fear death; I just wasn't ready to die. I still wanted to travel to Italy, and hoped to become a grandparent, although that, of course, wasn't in my control. Still, I hoped.

Whatever kind of seizures mine were, they left me unnerved and terror-stricken through January.

Already a pattern had emerged; each was more intense and longer in duration than the last. This realization caused me significant worry as I imagined hour-long seizures. Were there no treatments? Would there be no turning back from what appeared to be continuous physical and cognitive decline?

Dale continued recording short videos of seizures, as requested, except filming was usually interrupted by shared terror. And an instinctive need to dial 911.

~

I eagerly awaited the following Monday morning without patience or resilience, desperate to talk to my neurologist at the epilepsy clinic. I needed to be heard and believed. Can't they do something about these seizures and figure out a plan? Finally, discouragement and anger erupted.

Why was it taking so long to get support for whatever it was that was broken in me? Didn't they know that it's impossibly difficult to wait seven years?

I closed my eyelids, then felt like my rage needed an outlet. I slapped paint onto canvas and scraped my fingernails through the wet paint in a vain attempt to interpret my irritation, fear, and emotions. It felt difficult to label and express my emotions with words. It felt right to use hues of black and red, to let my emotions be sculpted into a texture of layers of acrylic and to fully immerse my hands in the process. It felt good, like the guilty pleasure of scraping your nails across a chalkboard that elicits a primal response. Painting my seizures was like a prehistoric warning call from my body as I created a petroglyph symbolizing my turbulent, out of control mind as it screamed, *Pay attention!*

~

It had been three hundred and forty-nine days since I'd welcomed students to a classroom. Three hundred forty-nine calendar days checked off on the calendar, which now hung in my home office rather than in a classroom or at a school. Three hundred forty nine days since students trusted me in a learning space I'd created.

I loved how they'd simultaneously challenged me with their "tough" questions. I never pretended to have all the answers as they hurled queries hoping to put their teacher on the hot seat. I wasn't the expert at anything but found delight in facilitating their learning. I missed their exuberance as we created, questioned, made messy mistakes, experienced failures, and learned alongside one another.

I missed those hallowed hallways through which inquisitive learners joyfully skipped and ran, even when they weren't supposed to. I longed to hear the spontaneous eruption of full-out belly laughter. I craved that satisfying feeling a teacher gets when a child shares that they love coming to school, knowing you've made a difference in their lives. Ironically, I even missed that brave space where students come to stand next to me or beside my desk, to fart, so astute classmates didn't dare giggle, point, or humiliate them. They were already embarrassed enough that they'd needed to pass gas and I'd prayed nobody else noticed. But someone always had.

Whenever there was an opportunity to support their

emotional needs, I'd tried to the best of my ability. That mattered to me, and still does. Vulnerable students require specialized supports. All children deserve care.

I was that kid, excited and unable to wait, wanting to be seen, heard, and understood. I longed for a wink of acknowledgment and wished to know that someone truly understood me. I longed until, what I'd been waiting for all along, was finally offered by a twenty-one-year-old, blue-eyed Swede, my Dale.

I was mischievous like our kids. They stayed up late by flashlight hiding under the covers caressing pages captivated by a story. I'd waited instead, willing myself to stay awake and for Mom to arrive home after a twelve-hour shift, hopeful that she'd give me a hug, and to hear "Goodnight, Jocelyn. I love you." That's what I'd wanted.

Our kids, I hoped would learn to anticipate and know they could count on both of us to speak their love language and return to scold because we cared enough. We'd return as many times as it took and say, "I love you, (insert name here), although I don't always love your behaviour. It's time to turn off your light, put your book away and sleep." Leaving, I'd lovingly plant one more kiss, to ensure they remember, as weary lids closed and as twinkling eyes awakened, that they were loved.

~

Tears flowed down my cheeks one Sunday night. I found myself suddenly sad, and wondered what had prompted these pearls of liquid, and why? I found myself ruminating about our now grown children, my past students and professional life. I'd lost people and things irretrievably. Things weren't as I expected.

Sunday nights had been when I thought about my students' vulnerabilities and needs as I planned for the week ahead. I missed being trusted with their secrets and burdens, and believed as an educator, who cared. I'd helped them carry their load and they, I was surprised to realize, mine. I missed all of it, every part about being a teacher.

I'd needed someone in 2014. I'd needed a community-of-care between 2014–2021 to reassure and reiterate that it would be okay to speak about sadness and express anger. I'd needed gentle reminders that suggested, considering the circumstances, it was normal and human nature to experience a wide range of emotions in the wake of traumatic incidents. There'd been too many.

I hoped there might be someone, or anyone, who'd see my needs and ask: How are you managing after this year's staffing process and the loss of your cherished teaching position?

I'd earned and held that position for five years as the best-qualified candidate, only to have it taken. Others listened as I vented then, nodded with empathy saying, "I understand." They didn't. They couldn't.

They hadn't been equipped with the just-right questions to ask, or supportive responses I'd required. I talked, but nobody noticed. If they did, perhaps they didn't think it polite to pry. If only they'd had the courage to observe and ask, then listen without trying to solve what ailed me.

I'd needed them to have had bravado when I did not. Even if just a little more. It would have been enough, and much more than I had.

In fact, I'd required supportive care and more during the Sixties, Seventies, and Eighties when I longed for someone to draw me in, reassure me I was safe and loved, and to hold me close. Perhaps then I'd have known I was lovable. That, I am lovable.

My body recognized, what I did not. That every "body" is unique, preordained, and gifted with resilience and self-determination. If only others had expressed a willingness to come alongside and sit with me in silence during difficult times. I'd been experiencing discomfort. For nearly five decades my body struggled to communicate what I didn't dare express aloud. My struggles were no one's fault; not mine or anyone else's.

I'd needed support I didn't have.

By 2021, molars and incisors gnashed metaphorically and literally. Teeth and tongue collided in defiance to publicly articulate perceived injustices. A fierce backlash developed as my body kept the score of unresolved grief and loss. Limbs and body ranted about offenses taken and iniquities that only my subconscious understood after it stored strong emotions I didn't dare utter.

I'd locked my heart up and safely forgotten where I'd tucked the only key. The one that might unlock an escape route to wellness.

I hadn't yet learned to listen to my body, nor had they listened to mine. And in the absence of physical evidence that might draw attention to what I'd safely secured, no one guessed my heart's secrets.

~

What made saying, "I love you, Jocelyn" so hard? I was angry and resentful at fifty-six, recognizing I'd never heard those words from a parent. I hadn't learned to prioritize self-care or to love myself. I had boundless empathy for others, though none in reserve for me. I sensed in vivid detail and with crippled emotions believed what I thought. As I empathized with others about what it might be like to watch me seize or be my caregiver, I forgot the importance that it was okay to not be okay and to express how I felt.

I didn't need to conjure shock or the stunned look of alarm on Dale's face to register how he might feel. Guilt informed me of the wreckage I'd caused as I gazed into Dale's now grey-blue eyes, aged as they'd witnessed a loved one's terror and pain without the ability to fix it. Shards and fragments of my lived experiences lay strewn like tossed litter after the fact and strained the individual resilience of too many who loved me deeply and supported me as I struggled for self-determination, clarity, and a diagnosis. My health exacted a cost that rippled out and affected loved ones, friends, and my community at large. Who knew the exponential impact of undiagnosed health?

~

There are not enough adequate words to describe what occurred Thursday, January 23, 2021. As the eighth seizure of the day began, I'd collapsed, like a wounded bird who hadn't sensed the glass and had flown directly into the windowpane.

The morning started out like any other post hump-day during an otherwise ordinary workweek. Except, I hadn't worked for almost a year. But then from sunrise to sunset, I seized. I'd long remember this date as momentous, and perhaps worthy of scrapbooking, if I cared to remember details already etched on my soul.

Jealously guarded emotions, like long-jailed captives released from chains during a riot, wreaked havoc and seized that day. They erupted from behind reinforced steel bars and fled confinement as they zigged and zagged creating pandemonium.

Legs cursed, jaws collided, and prisoners rattled tin cups on steel bars. Fueled by inert energy long silenced, body parts stiffened by stored misfortune and drama, it cut loose. As the first seizure of the day climaxed, I'd found myself face to face, or hands to face, with the warden. Uncontrollable rage clamped airways shut and released anger needing escape broke free.

~

I'd turned to tell Dale. "There's tingling in my cheeks." I sat up, thinking it might be easier to inhale more deeply that way. I presumed it might also relieve the pain I was experiencing behind my left eye. I was confused and thought I needed more air. I'd taught students when we'd practiced mindfulness in the classroom, that by extending the length of your exhale you can calm your worries. But my lizard brain had already taken over.

I filled my lungs with a deep inhale and believed if I could just get enough air, the light-headedness might subside. I was wrong.

I brought my hands to my face to show Dale where the spine-tingling prickles occurred. Then, without notice, my palms and fingers clasped my cheekbones and stuck. They pushed and slid inward, squishing my mouth into goldfish lips and covered my face, from the top of my eyebrows to under my chin, cocooning and covering both my nose and mouth.

Eyes, as if clothed by a skin-tight pair of jeans, sought Dale in terror.

Eyes, which couldn't see because they were unexpectedly wrapped over by fingers terrorizing rather than playfully asking, "Guess who?"

Dale intervened, *Thank God*, and forcibly removed my hands from covering airways. He peeled away each of my fingers from an undeniable attempt to smother and extinguish. Hands and digits received mixed messages from a once intelligent brain.

There'd been another siren. *I'm the one, this time.*

Instead of hearing and knowing someone else was in distress, buckled inside a speeding ambulance with its siren screeching and lights flashing, as I stopped to pray.

*Lord, please be with the paramedics, and the individual being rushed to the ER. You know their name, their needs, and love each of us. Prepare the hands and hearts of the medical professionals with discernment and knowledge, so that they'll be prepared to offer your healing and hope. Amen.*

Instead, this time, they were coming for me. AGAIN.

I was that somebody!

Throughout the day there were repetitive seizures of varied lengths. Airways opened and closed and couldn't conceal uncontrollable rage.

Eyes, opened wide, tried in vain to communicate.

*I can't breathe!*

Resolution came only when an instinctual will to live caused an involuntary gasp, and I'd sucked in air through oxygen starved airways.

Fear was my constant companion. As I'd nod off in a recliner, stood at the stove considering a cup of tea, or sat immune-compromised visiting with friends or ladies over Zoom for a bible study. Circumstances didn't seem to matter, as seizures started. They'd begin again and again. By mid-month, I'd sensed them coming as my head started to rock and I'd gasp for breath while my voice embedded itself in a body without volume. Sometimes, my fingers weren't claw-like, and I'd snap my fingers to alert Dale. Often, I could not.

*SNAP. SNAP. SNAP.*

Usually close by, I'd seek his reassuring presence. Clarity and knowledge were no longer allies, and answers hadn't appeared yet on the horizon.

Again... it would begin.

*What do you do but pray!*

Hearing snapping fingers from across the room Dale, a Godsend, arrived time and time again as the fingers on my right went rigid, crimped, and crooked, as if wired to create an armature for something prehistoric at the museum. The fingers of my left followed suit, in a game of cat and mouse. Arms and elbows spastically jerked with palatable violence and joined the party. They'd be no more, "Snap" or snapping.

I knew that during an epileptic seizure that it was possible to bite your tongue and feared it would happen to me. I valued my taste buds, willed my jaws to stop crashing and my tongue to seek shelter at the roof of my mouth. My limbs opened and closed, switched direction, and frequently ticked as if my body sheltered a bomb counting down.

Then, I felt pain and knew that my tongue had inadvertently got in the way. Instinct drew it in and up and later it felt bruised though had not drawn blood.

Vehement anger embedded in my inmost parts, extended its wrath from a place I couldn't control. Anger moved me as if I were a marionette manipulated by a demonic puppeteer.

The recliner, rocked across the floor. Not, gently as if to rock a baby to sleep, instead, violently without the use of an arm or a lever. My body manipulated the chair with its own life force and without nitrous oxide to propel it forward. I felt it break as one movement climaxed, and then another disorganized and convulsive movement began.

Dale timed… and I'd hear another ambulance streaking and squealing to the finish line. I'd run another a marathon.

Their first questions were always the same. This time answered by Keith, who filled in the blanks while Dale, first on the scene, comforted me. He'd only moved out of the way for the paramedic to move in and assess.

Keith detailed, and Dale added embellishments. "She has a history of seizures," I heard them say.

I listened, while my cheek rested on the carpet and my eyelids remained closed. I was spent. They told the extended version, and I wondered if it were me telling my story, how I might explain my seizures differently.

Keith and Dale were all facts and explained that I had a comprehensive team of neurologists in Vancouver, that I'd been waitlisted for "urgent" admission to the seizures investigation unit (SIU), and, "No, my neurologist didn't want them to give me Ativan."

Days filled with certainty of seizures and sleepless nights persisted as I waited for my mid-February "urgent" admission. Fifteen minutes became my marker of whether I'd have a seizure as I fell asleep at night, or not. If I could just get through those first fifteen, odds were increased that I'd have a peaceful rest. Tension built nightly as I brushed my teeth, as we filled CPAP tanks and turned off our reading lights. Bedtime, once a magical routine shared with Keith and Kristen, became a dreaded end of day ritual of bedtime seizures. As the sun set, my anxiety would rise and blind the moon with its intensity and brilliance.

~

Alone, each seizure might be troubling; together, they added up to endless terror. I was bound it seemed in a weave of sticky threads: stress, triggers, anxiety, compulsive behaviors, and anticipation of what appeared to be epileptic events. What once was unexpected, I could now safely assume would occur without making an ass of myself.

My emotions, likewise, were as tangled as my hair after an extended EEG. It would take a whole bottle of conditioner to tame those tangles, knots which now gripped me. I needed a new and improved formula that would both detangle and de-stress a frazzled mind, while I waited for the puppeteer to release the strings and admit me to the SIU.

# CHAPTER NINETEEN

**Who Holds Your Heart – An Unorthodox Rerun**

I'd recognized grief and loss, and that they'd been leaking from the inside out. Dale hadn't been able to cure what ailed me, as amazing as he was, and Valentine's Day seemed as distant as Mars. Could I survive the six weeks, or until an admission date to the seizures investigation unit (SIU) was confirmed? My faith in God was strengthening out of necessity.

Each morning I headed into my home office after Dale left for work to center myself and pray. Some days were more difficult than others, as I passed through the door and seated myself. It was hard to have such a weighted list of needs to lift.

I'd read a daily devotional and listened to one of a few favourite playlists I'd created. I wanted to begin each day with gratitude. Even when I'd struggled, which had been most days, I'd chosen to make this prayer time a priority. It grounded me at a time I expected to have daily seizures, chronic back pain, and a weakened core.

Long January days filled with bizarre, repetitive movements and sitting for long periods recovering from seizures, combined with a lack of physical activity, left me desperate and alone.

I needed to rehearse movements mentally and physically before attempting to stand, after sitting, and before walking. I couldn't stand unsupported, or walk for more than six minutes without having a seizure, as the discouraging days of January dropped as if sand through an hourglass.

After I'd completed my daily devotional on January 25, I'd organized my core, and mentally checked that muscles were prepared and ready, before standing and heading to the washroom across the hall. I'd been humming a worship tune as I left what once had been Kristen's bedroom and was now my home office. Not remembering all the lyrics, I hummed the chorus.

*"I surrender all, I surrender all. All to Thee, My blessed Savior. I surrender all."* The tune brought forth a smile I noticed in my mirrored reflection as I passed by the bathroom mirror and mindfully stopped to consider whether to shower and wash my hair.

Then this had happened.

My gaze softened, shoulders fell, and I'd released my grip from one of two grab bars, which doubled as towel racks. Dale had special ordered and installed five grab bars in our main, upstairs bathroom, needed to ensure my safety. Without a conscious awareness I began to sing the words of the song I'd been humming.

Walls and furniture had become touch points I'd required in 2017, to stand unsupported. I'd been unable to organize my core and use both hands simultaneously to blow dry my hair or pour boiling water from the kettle into a tea pot through 2020. By 2021, I'd needed Dale's arm and bodily strength for support.

As I sang the hymn, I lifted willing hands, which propelled themselves upward as I closed my eyes. Minutes passed before recognition dawned, and I realized that the rooted soles of my bare feet were parallel and about six inches apart. They'd supported me. *Or had they?* Perhaps, I'd leaned into trust, and not on my own understanding.

Standing unsupported hadn't been possible for the better part of four years. A photograph, I thought, would remind me that without thought or effort I'd lifted willing hands and surrendered and then rejoiced with gratitude.

From deep inside me the song arose as if it had its own heartbeat, and the lyrics I'd needed were provided, as my soul soaked up healing light for all the dark crevices. The well of my soul had been nourished with living water, rather than depleted by mixed-up messages and error codes which hissed along neural pathways in disguise. God had calmed the storm.

Still in my cotton polka-dotted nightie I wanted to capture a photo keepsake, which would capture the essence of this flash of insight. I zipped to the kitchen, retrieved my phone, and recreated the scene, which captured the space between the patterned dots and navy trimmed hem of my nightie and the patterned linoleum where my feet had been. Only my toes peeked out from beneath the dark blue hem.

I held the phone with its 12-megapixel camera, steadying it against my body facing straight down and captured a bird's eye view of both my feet and in the background my favourite purple and grey Haflinger wool clogs. Like a ballerina's slippers they'd been cast off in the shadow of the countertop and rested in first position.

God met me there.

I hadn't dared to move a muscle or take a step, as I savoured this gift. Minutes passed as I stood and sang. It was wonderous, and upon reflection, perhaps miraculous.

~

Time and time again, I returned to writing and art, which like prayers flowed through me as I waited for admission to the SIU. I'd been reassured that the admission would happen sometime in the next six weeks early in January. Though I'd prayed it would sometime soon.

At one of many extreme lows there'd been a particular string of bad days that kicked me to the curb. That's when I'd needed and had drawn creative inspiration after learning mindfulness exercises led by an inspired art therapist to release my grief and losses. These sessions with paints in hand had been an opportunity to get out of my head and to allow my body to choose the colours to express itself.

After those first complex seizures in early January, I'd squeezed acrylic hues from four-ounce plastic tubes: black, red, and purple onto a cookie sheet, then pinned and hung vertically four pieces of plain chart paper. Together, they'd created a gigantic three-foot-wide rectangular canvas.

With the knowledgeable support of an art therapist, I'd allowed unwanted thoughts to glide by, and instead listened to my body as I portrayed the seizures I'd experienced. I'd painted blackened swaths with wispy tails, scraped fingers dipped in scarlet acrylic dripping with anger, and created a dark-faced, winged apparition who appeared to have been silenced by the presence of a charred black speech bubble.

I later wondered if perhaps my soul fled my body amidst the smudged spatters and reddish-purple blood-stained painted scrapes. Had something imprisoned, escaped? Could I tell you what it all meant as I'd stood back to reflect afterwards?

No.

Could I explain why I'd chosen the colours my fingers knew to pick up and squeeze onto the cookie sheet?

No, again.

It hadn't been an intellectual pursuit.

I sponged paint marbled with both black and red on to the canvas, and later thought, that the shapes were coffin-like. They appeared to frame the chaos they bound. This was only the first of three blank canvases I painted January 4, 2021.

I had more to say, more pain and more fear to process and not enough paper, even after I covered nine square feet. Each canvas told a different story.

I continued to paint what would be the second of three paintings, as anger leaked from my pores. Was I a caged lioness willing her release? Fury expressed itself with urgency, after seizures, and demanded a pardon.

The second painting, this time created on the right side of my 14" x 17" coil-bound sketchbook began with broad blood-red ribbons of acrylic. The surface became a place where imprisoned pain and guarded emotions were shelved for future contemplation.

I thrust hands into sprawling blobs and swept fingers again cloaked in scarlet across the page. Without cleaning my hands, I re-dipped them in what had been midnight black and dark purple acrylic. Without defined edges or curves to differentiate each hue after painting the first large canvas, I added layered handprints scattered over the surface.

As if a kid in kindergarten, without a large enough piece of paper, I'd extended the release of pain onto a third page. I pressed palms and fingers, joints, and creases, into now multicoloured blobs and added colour to the third of what would become a trio of representative artwork.

Looking back, I noticed that I'd created photographic replicas of my hands with their time-etched lines, creases, and scars with the varied shades of purple and black.

Handprints, like the motley bruises that had showed up after each blown IV attempt at the ER. Nurses and paramedics had taken well-intentioned stabs and hurried attempts to properly thread each IV needle to find a vein that would work. Many of the attempts had caused reddish-purple bruises up and down my forearms on more than one occasion.

"You're a hard target," they often commented in the emergency room. Small veins, poor hydration, and primal fear aren't a great combination when being admitted to the ER for URGENT care, as I'd been numerous times.

Later, I washed my hands in hot soapy water prepared earlier contained in a recycled ice-cream pail and double-checked to ensure there'd not been residual paint embedded under my fingernails, or on my forearms. On occasion, I found dried swatches of flaky colour on my skin, missed during cleanup. I became more conscientious and cleaned with extra vigour. I needed to get it right, in a landscape where it seemed I controlled nothing.

Each handprint left a story imprinted in acrylic and

consequently an opportunity to reflect on events through varied lenses. I believed the paintings were finished.

I washed up and then realized, they weren't.

There'd been a tug and I was pulled to reconsider. Were embellishments needed, my intellect asked. Were my perfectionism and desire to get it right, speaking, or had it been my heart that hinted the trio were incomplete?

Reaching over to the cubby where I stored various tubes of acrylic beside my art table, I gave my heart and hands permission to be guided to one last colour, gold.

My body had chosen hues which epitomized emotional distress, and its dysregulation. As I stood back, I was prompted to notice what was missing, and to add one last hue.

The urgency of waiting escalated with each seizure. Would it really take specialists almost two months to get to the Klondike, strike it rich and hit pay dirt, before I'd be able to head to the SIU? I'd experienced three seizures, then eight in a single day. *Was I going to be able to get through this? What would provide me with the prerequisite strength and armour?*

~

I pressed both hands, first right then left, into yellow gold. My body rather than my brain guided the process. I rolled both palms and fingers in the godlike hue and created fingerprints, like facial recognition ID for a laptop or smart phone.

I lifted and rested my fingers in the paint repeatedly. In this way I ensured every inch of skin on both hands sparkled. I left metallic-textured handprints to layer, cover, and provide much needed protection against what weighed me down.

His Spirit, in me, had stamped its living presence on each of the pages and paintings. They'd been permanently tattooed, lest I forget I'd been chosen as His Beloved. I signed and dated the trio of newly created images.

Then, exhaled.

~

The vague suggestion that it might be mid-February

before I was admitted for further investigation caused hopelessness. It seemed ages away and things were getting worse. The Calvary didn't seem to be coming, and I was getting more and more desperate.

Making and creating had become life-giving tools that breathed hope into days I'd been overwhelmed by seizures, struggled to breathe, and discouraged. I'd written a poem after I'd painted, which I later titled, "Surrender."

My fear of death had been calmed, and I'd begun to innately sense God's protection. It hadn't occurred to me then, that my poem would become my prayer:

*Spirit, lead me to surrender to a place of calm with a spirit of trust.*
*Quiet, my anxious spirit.*
*Strengthen my quickening, beating heart.*
*Stamp your living presence in my every part, and quiet my mind. It's time for rest.*
*Like handprints with a protective gold shield, refine me, and make me whole.*
*With your living presence, mark and claim me, that I will remember and believe that you*
*delight in me, and love unconditionally.*
*Help me, Jesus. Fill me with your Peace.*
*Show me Your Ways.*
*Amen.*

~

I looked in the rear view mirror fearfully those next five days, instead of ahead to where my Heavenly Father stood beckoning. I walked anxiously under my own steam with only early childhood's learned responses to light the way.

Only on occasion, had I been able to claim His protection and calm myself when I was injured, afraid or hurt. I discounted God's omniscience, omnipotence, and unconditional love during most of 2020, and through the early weeks of the new year.

Self-control, it had seemed, was better than no control.

And I'd been blinded by terror and despair. Had I neglected to remember that He'd been beside me all along.

~

There'd been a lone hummingbird who came to our feeder throughout an uncharacteristic deep freeze in the Comox Valley, when temperatures had fallen to minus seven degrees Celsius, or six Fahrenheit, the winter of 2020-21. He'd come to feed year-round from the transparent plastic cylinder I'd filled repeatedly with a ruby sugar-water solution. At times, he perched to feed. Alternately, with his needle-like beak perfect for reaching he'd fed himself with his specialized tongue that grabbed and trapped the artificial homemade nectar before carrying the sought-after liquid into his mouth. It was an adequate solution, that meet his needs, when nectar from suitable flowers hadn't been available.

His presence made me smile during the cold wet-weather months on Vancouver Island and had been an exceptionally relevant reminder. He'd been willing to accept nurture and nourishment through months when brightly coloured, tubular-shaped, red blooms had vanished. He taught me, it was okay not to be okay.

~

It became apparent during one of my lowest of lows that I'd needed to cede control and ask for help. I no longer had the required capacities to manage or control my chaotic life. I tried to surrender my fears and trust to God, however it was a struggle I wrestled for control over. I fought to survive against a tyrannical inner critic, with a fragile psyche and hadn't won.

I implored God, seeking, and surrendering throughout January. Finally, I believed He alone could meet my spiritual needs. I recognized my desire to reclaim gifts that had been freely offered and already given. His presence provided me self-determination, wisdom, and guidance to mature in my faith and strengthened me to practice radical self-acceptance and, most importantly, trust.

Confidence and assertiveness weren't skills I was well

versed in and were still blurred edges to the trust I offered others. And especially to Dale, who, I believed, I'd trusted all along. I'd stopped seeking heavenly guidance and when God had called me out upon the waters or into the great unknown, I floundered like Peter. He found and sheltered me during this period of unbelief and still called me by name.

I aimed to trust when seizures overtook me, my brain made mistakes, and as my body seized, but failed. I had fierce survival instincts, and my reptilian brain took over, as I fled to a secret safe place and escaped the terror.

I had a little faith and wanted more.

Lord, hear my voice. "Out of the depths, I have cried to You, O Lord!" (Psalm 130)

~

I documented seizures on blustery January days as I peered out the window and witnessed above average amounts of rainfall, sleet, or snow, dependent on the daily temperatures. Precipitation brought courtesy of La Niña to the southwest portion of British Columbia, while humankind entered a second year of pandemic protocols.

Seizures and events, inscribed, jerked, and stamped themselves on my being at a time when I was already under the influence of post-traumatic stress. I hadn't known or been able to control toxic shame, abject feelings of loneliness, or the learned, hair-trigger fight/flight response my brain had normalized.

Had I subconsciously summoned an artist to ink the regressions? Had my body learned to speak and describe emotional flashbacks that lacked a visual translation? I hadn't remembered any noteworthy childhood incidents, when the psychiatrist had asked, or much of anything prior to the age of four.

Had the cognitive impairment documented just before Christmas in 2020, been the result of seizures, as they'd suggested? Or was my poor memory due to some other, yet undiagnosed, life-threatening illness? I was in a desperate state and there was still four weeks plus a day to wait. Would the seven-year wait, become seventy? Would I live that long?

Hues twisted across the page as pain illustrated unmet needs, and my body created images that signaled grief and loss. Seizures, like oxygen-hungry tissues expressed their need for arterial blood and spoke up. They conveyed my brain's inability to send and receive well-articulated messages through neural pathways.

*Dearest Jesus, am I ever going to get the call, and be admitted?*

~

I'd hoped that I might recover my ability to relax, provide self-care, and eliminate my harsh self-critic, but instead of motherly warmth and words of affection through 2020, I continued to be my mother's care-partner while exponentially increasing complex seizures uprooted my life.

Instead of steroid injections of a pharmaceutical biologic, like Rituximab, when they'd thought I had seronegative autoimmune encephalitis in 2020, I'd needed infusions of parental love to be fortified in the 1960s, when at four I'd required hugs, reassurances I was safe, and to hear words of affection.

And again, in January 2021, I needed a fully functioning parent, rather than a dependent with dementia. I missed Mom's presence and still longed for a parent to comfort me tenderly.

Each unexpected rhythmic jerk, I'd believed, could be the start of a life-threatening event those last weeks of January. There'd been some unverified evidence that this wasn't the case; however, my child-like psyche catalogued each intensified seizure with fear and uncertainty.

~

I'd knocked at the door as a child in Sunday School, again at a teen retreat, and at various other times when I struggled. And again, at thirty when I'd become a first-time parent with a newborn in my arms. Had He answered? He had. Had I trusted?

Faith isn't an easy journey, however it's knowing that you need help, and that you're held, that makes the difference.

I'd still not heard back from my epileptologist with a confirmed admission date those last days of January. With only sixteen calendar days remaining till the estimated admissions date of mid-February my seizures were getting worse, much worse. The clock was barely ticking. Was I doomed to be stuck in this hellish season of agony endlessly?

~

I'd walked alone in self-determination. Without a friendly manager of my psyche to signal that I needed to prioritize self-compassion and preservation. I'd believed myself an imposter throughout my career, despite continuous accolades for professional accomplishments. Was I wasting everyone's time, energy, and resources? Was I an imposter and liar, as one doctor and another had implied? I worried that the time would come and that I'd surely be discovered as the fraud I knew myself to be. I'd simply been faking it until I could make it. I hadn't made it yet.

Could all these physical symptoms, and seizures be in my head?

I knew they weren't, but I was so crazy messed up from the waiting, uncertainty, and seizures, that I'd unknowingly given others permission to get in my head and had begun to doubt my intelligence and worth.

Seizures were distractions, which vied for my attention. Had I regressed and become a child, at fifty-seven? A naïve, honest, yet ill-equipped adult, who continued to lack emotional maturity and failed to complete numerous important developmental tasks due to environmental, rather than genetically caused, influences in childhood?

I'd forgotten to whom I belonged, that I'd been gifted a lamp to light the way, and that I had a trusted guide to show the way.

After my biological father disappeared in 1966, I struggled without emotional resilience, while my beloved mother nurtured with a disposition of fear and anxiety due to her own repressed needs. She hadn't realized I required her to express affection. She'd done the best she could, which was enough to keep me physically secure. However, I hadn't thrived without the security and safety of hearing and believing I was loved and held.

Somewhere along the way, I imagined and stepped into God's role. I naively believed I met the required qualifications. Through the Seventies, Eighties, and Nineties, I wished silently upon a star that I'd be able to stay in each newly decorated bedroom, remain at the same school for a second year in a row, or to enter the seventh grade and be among the eldest and most capable senior students in a K–7th grade elementary school. I hoped to keep that dream job as our district's itinerant gifted education teacher, teaching gifted learners. Instead, I learned that wishing upon a star hadn't helped. I'd been laid-off annually for almost a decade, and then again after five years in a permanent contract. It had been time to pray instead of wishing, so in 2021, I'd prayed.

~

I paused after creating each painted depiction that cried out from the depths of me. There'd been sorrow, pain, and intensity in what I painted after seizures. When I prayed, most often my prayers were only desperate pleas. I tried to let my ears be attentive. I cried out in paralyzing grief. *Hear me! Hear my groans! Hear my cry amidst the depths.* (Psalm 61:1, Psalm 130:1-8) I'd longed for God to hear my requests and turn his ear to me. I couldn't bear to remain in this season of perpetual wallowing in the depths. I prayed each morning, lifted my needs, and waited expectantly. In His word, I hoped.

*Hear my cry for help, my King, and my God, for to you I pray.* (Psalm 5:1-2)

My hope had been nothing more than a warm optimism. Each time I repeated my prayer of surrender, taken a posture of confident expectation and entrusted my future to Him,

I hoped in God as an act of faith. Then I foolishly took back what I lifted. I doubted like Thomas, a skeptic who refused to believe without direct personal experience. Except, I witnessed miracles and still not trusted. I lacked bravery to navigate as I cried out from the depths.

I waited throughout January for God to meet me. Unlike Ezekiel, who'd been commissioned to keep watch while he'd waited for the morning, I surrendered control and hoped what little faith I did have would be enough. While I waited, I seized.

Whether or not I'd been aware, He'd held me each time.

~

February broadcast the climax of Mt. Washington's snowpack for outdoor winter enthusiasts, and the arrival of Groundhog Day. At sea level in the Town of Comox, we enjoyed two and three day stretches of sunshine between periods of cooler temperatures and overcast skies.

Events triggered thoughts that prompted mixed emotions. I experienced fear for my life, health, and well-being and sadness caused by a repetitive cycle of each event seeming worse than the last. I believed I was powerless over my seizures and cognitive decline. Guilt triggered thoughts that I was the cause of my family's distress, and that somehow my actions were to blame.

Anger expressed itself, though I was unaware, as goals I valued and prioritized were blocked, interrupted, or prevented. Together this perfect storm of emotions left me feeling that I was being personally attacked, and that I needed to fight, freeze, flee or fawn.

However, love prevailed. Even on days and nights when I experienced seizures, I was offered and gifted things I needed: by God, Dale, and the actions of family, friends, colleagues, students, and neighbours, which sparked sentimentality, tenderness, and warmth.

Through the first ten days of February, as always, Dale ensured I knew he still saw me as both smart and attractive. His words and actions were constant reminders that he hadn't changed his mind since he'd vowed, "I do!"

I continued to be overwhelmed by the reduced quality of my life. However, because of Dale who'd point at me with invisible eyebrows lifted and grin before bursting into song, I was able to smile.

"I'm looking for a smart woman in a real short skirt." Then he changed the lyrics to: "I've got a smart woman, who knows how to flirt."

Time, and again I was healed by his words of affection. Dale was my joy-bringer, confidant, and strongest advocate during this, and every other season. Especially during what was one of the most difficult seasons when I didn't love myself.

Whether I was aware or blindly wandered, Dale's presence and love infiltrated the darkest crevices of me, and I knew, I was blessed. A seed of hope had been planted, God provided the seed and the sower, and Dale nurtured and ensured it was sown in fertile ground. He gave me the support and courage to grow and bear fruit, which gave me courage. I was mightily blessed.

"Lord, I cry out to you from the depths of my life. Hurt, confusion, and sorrow fill me... But I can stand because there is forgiveness with You... My future is securely in Your hands. Thus, may I hope."

I was in serious trouble, Dale was freaking the hell out on the inside, and neither of us were excited to celebrate my February birthday, only days away. We shared a singular focus as we waited for a call that would confirm an admission date to the SIU.

Dale was hopeful the morning of February 10; I was overwhelmed. That afternoon... the phone rang.

# PART FOUR

## SEASON OF CLARITY

JOCELYN BYSTROM

# CHAPTER TWENTY

## The Call

Friday, February 12, 2021, I was expected, at last.

My neurologist had phoned January 10, late in the day, after I'd heard from the clerk at Vancouver General Hospital's seizures investigation unit. Always thorough, Dr. Percy wanted to confirm that I had received the date and necessary details from the admissions clerk. She knew I'd need to hear her steadying voice. She was right.

I thanked her for her compassion and reassurances. Then, she implied that it was critical to my mental health that I heed the following advice: "Bring lots of things to entertain yourself at the SIU, and your favourite snacks." Others had found themselves literally bored stiff waiting endless hours day after day for seizures, while they'd been restricted to being seated or lying in bed. I had easily imagined being fenced into the 40 x 80 inch rectangular cell that would be my bed. I'd had only one previous neurology admission, but a visit to the SIU would be altogether different.

"Some patients," she'd said, "are admitted to the SIU, wait three weeks, only to be sent home without results after not having had a single seizure."

I didn't believed that would be my problem, since I'd had at least one, if not multiple seizures, every day for the past week.

My takeaways from her sage advice:

1) Be prepared to entertain yourself twenty-four seven,.

2) *Wait, what?* It was possible to end up going home *without* a diagnosis? That wasn't reassuring.

~

It had been hurry up and wait for nearly seven years, and now the evening of February 10, knowing we'd be leaving in the morning, suddenly I needed more time.

*What does one pack for a three-week stint to the SIU?*

It wouldn't be like packing for a typical vacation. I wouldn't need my swimsuit, the mandatory item I always packed first in my overnight bag. There hadn't been time for me to receive a "What to Expect" brochure, so I spread items I thought I might need, or simply wanted, across the queen-sized bed in our guest room. The strange assortment covered the duvet, awaiting decisions that I felt ill-equipped to make.

The admissions clerk, who'd called from the SIU, suggested I bring only tops that either zipped or buttoned.

"It's okay for you to wear your own comfortable clothes," she'd reassured. I was thrilled not to have to wear hospital garb. "But nothing that requires being pulled over your head," she reiterated.

I'd be in bed for up to twenty-one days, while neurology, respirology, and psychiatric teams waited for seizures, collected evidence, and collaborated to determine a diagnosis.

Reading my mind, the admission clerk had offered, "You'll be able to shower once a week."

Every seven days? I was horrified. Had I heard correctly? My daily routine at home included stepping into the tub, pulling the shower curtain across the rail, adjusting the temperature, and then reaching for the handheld shower wand soon after my feet hit the ground. I couldn't imagine a week without a shower.

Okay, I told myself, pack comfy clothes:
- Fleece pajama bottoms and stretchy footless tights, like the kind you

typically wear under a dress, or long tunic-styled sweater.
- Socks. I'd need those to keep my feet toasty. But how many pairs?
- And slippers? Would I need slippers? Maybe not, if I couldn't leave the bed. But surely, I would be up out of bed to use the washroom. I wasn't an invalid.

The clerk from the SIU had also anticipated this question, and thoughtfully filled in all the blanks.

*Hmm, tops?* As I hunted through dresser drawers and my closet, I realized that I didn't have an abundance, or even a few, of the appropriate button up or zip up shirts and blouses. Apparently, I preferred tops and sweaters that stretched and pulled over my noggin. I didn't think to sensibly raid Dale's side of the closet.

Late in the day, I walked down Comox Avenue and headed downtown to see what I could locate mid-pandemic. I passed one and then another thrift shop, each displaying closed until further notice signs. These were not uncommon to see in storefront windows, in January 2021, in the Comox Valley. Shops hadn't yet reopened since closing their doors early in the pandemic when the world collectively held its breath.

I only found one upscale ladies wear store open for business downtown. Perhaps they'd have something appropriate on a sale rack. The door to the shop was already open, with a posted sign requiring customers to wear masks and use hand sanitizer prior to entry. It also stated the store's capacity limit: *2 Customers at a time, PLEASE!*

I leaned in through the opened doorway to gauge who, if any, were already inside. Two customers max isn't many, perhaps only a couple.

"Do you have any button up shirts, or blouses on your sale rack?" I asked from the entryway, without entering. And then as an afterthought added, "Anything that doesn't need to be pulled over your head."

I was hesitant to enter the store to check price tags while still immunocompromised from steroid infusions, and after being told that my first vaccine from a few weeks earlier may only provide 50 percent effectiveness.

The store's clerk returned with a single possibility, a navy blouse. "I'll take it," I said, without even asking the cost; there were no other options.

~

February 11 was travel day for Kristen and me. I hugged and kissed Dale goodbye, which wasn't easy. We'd discussed and agreed that he'd needed to stay home and work. He planned to video chat with me daily.

Besides, even if he travelled with me to Vancouver, he'd only be allowed to visit briefly during limited visiting hours, once each day. And I'd only be allowed one visitor per day. We'd talked it over and decided Kristen could be my visitor during the workweek and Dale would travel to Vancouver the following Friday, as my weekend visitor. It made sense but was tough leaving my #1 encourager and best friend behind.

Kristen and I headed out to Vancouver General's SIU, where I'd encounter the great unknown, alone.

# CHAPTER TWENTY-ONE

### Hoping for Seizures

I was on an emotional roller coaster between hope and terror. What was wrong with me? What was going to happen next? What if these guys couldn't figure it out? God's providential care didn't always seem aligned with my thoughts. I had a little faith and wanted more.

I entered the private room following a nurse from the SIU's admissions desk and was immediately aware of eau de antiseptic. It wasn't the Hilton. There were no chocolates left on my pillow. Instead, the bed rail was lowered, and the waiting was over.

February 12, 2021, had finally arrived and I hoped for answers.

I masked fear with a clever disguise, hopefulness.

Who hasn't headed straight to their computer and an online search engine after the first hint of a frightening diagnosis?

Historically, there were some scary treatments thought to cure seizures. *One Flew Over the Cuckoo's Nest* coloured an entire generation's perception, and mine, about the use of electroconvulsive therapy, better known as electric shock therapy, to treat seizures. Supposed cures they believed would promote changes in how brain cells communicated with each other and restore healthy brain function. Was ECT still used to treat epilepsy? I was pretty sure the answer was no, but needed to be reassured So, I'd Googled, before the admission.

If they couldn't stop my seizures or figure out what caused them, then what? Was I going to be okay?

Once you've gone down the rabbit hole it's hard to come up for air. I read about Hippocrates, in fifth century BC, who rejected the idea that epilepsy was caused by evil spirits, who set the blood in motion and caused seizures to be suffered by those with unstable or low morals, as the Catholic Church at the time believed. *Really?* I thought.

Hippocrates proposed that epilepsy was not divine in origin, and instead a medically treatable problem originating in the brain. If I had epilepsy, would it be treatable? Then again, maybe I didn't have epilepsy. They'd ruled out brain tumors, cancer, MS, and Parkinson's disease. If not epilepsy, would those be back on the table?

I wanted to get off this demonic coaster and have my life back, that's what I needed. I stretched out on my new bed knowing I would soon be tethered by wires and electrodes and unable to physically flee. I signed up for this, hoped for this.

Dr. Percy had implied that three weeks could feel like an eternity when you're tethered to your bed—by the head, no less. I'd recalled scenes from Hollywood thrillers, when captives were chained by their ankles to a metal bed with only a thin mattress and a single blanket. Scenes where hostages crouched in the dark, in dreary underground locations desperate for heroic rescue. They'd hug themselves while curled in the fetal position. *I've been waiting with bated breath for this.*

*What the hell was I thinking?*

Dr. Percy, my epileptologist, played a pivotal role in my seizure's investigation being expedited, and I knew it was the correct plan. It seemed like a good idea, right up until I arrived.

I was calm, *kind of*, when I was able to stop unwanted thoughts and listened to soothing instrumental worship music.

In those moments before I emptied my suitcase and clutched treasured items to remind me of God's provision of a safe place of stillness, fear oozed out like sunscreen and covered my thoughts. I needed to remind myself again and again that I was exactly where I belonged, and in expert hands. Held.

All would be well. I knew my family and friends were praying for my healing and recovery. I tried to remember and trust God's infinite mercy when I had a reflex to panic. Would I be able to remember as I seized? I hoped so.

I tried not to catastrophize or question, but....

*But* negated and cancelled out my faith whenever I seized. It stripped my soul of trust and much-needed calm.

*Would the first seizure be before or after I was settled and ready?*

I emptied my suitcase and strategically placed each item into the tall boy nightstand on wheels with one shallow and two deep drawers. Nerves settled as I touched familiar textures and comforting belongings, then raced when I contemplated scary diagnostic outcomes.

I carried my jacket, emptied suitcase, and clothes that needed hanging to the far corner of the room and hanging locker. A locker, like the one I'd had in high school, except taller, wider, and made of fiberboard. I hoisted the case for my CPAP machine on to the upper shelf, hung my jacket and wedged my suitcase into the perfectly sized space in the lower part of the locker. This suited my need to have everything in its place.

With the closet door closed my belongings would be out of the staff's way, and not pose a tripping hazard. I found "just right" places for most of what I brought, then stacked the rest of my belongings on the window ledge, not knowing where else to put them.

The last item packed was the first to be taken out. My

electric heating pad was a necessity for my chronically sore back and body. After finding an outlet to plug it in, I slipped the heating pad between the hospital-provided blanket and the favourite pillow I'd brought from home. I prepped my bed for much more than sleep. I even brought my own blankets and a quilt from home. I was going to be there for twenty-one days, twenty-four seven, and was anxious to ensure I was adequately prepared.

I came determined and ready.

~

From my room there was a view towards Vancouver's dense downtown core and the North Shore Mountains. A spectacle of glass-sided office towers filled the frame.

Looking down I noticed a rooftop maintenance area and multiple heat exchangers that dispersed steam. A rising cylindrical plume of grey streamed from each of the stacks. And like hospital operations, I presumed, would be operational twenty-four hours a day.

Hebrews 4:15 reminded me that my greatest hope in despair was the knowledge that the Son of God lived in flesh and empathized with my weakness. I hadn't wanted to be obedient to death, like Jesus was. I knew I couldn't manage that kind of pain. When terror struck during a seizure, I couldn't utter a prayer. If I had, it might have been: "Help me, Jesus!"

Standing at the window I wondered how lovely it might be if I were here in spring. I noticed not one, but two upper branches of what must be a tree with many life rings, and later learned that it might be one of many tulip trees, located along 10th Avenue. A tree that could reach heights of nearly seventy meters. I couldn't tell if the one I saw from my fifth floor window grew from the ground or from a pot on an unseen rooftop. Mid-February, there were only a couple of leaves that still clung to these upper branches. Bare limbs reached heavenward seeking, like me.

In those few precious moments before getting into bed for the duration, I stood by the window and savoured the view.

I wanted to be aware of the passage of time outside in the everyday world, which felt as distant as Dale in Comox, despite being only inches away outside the glass.

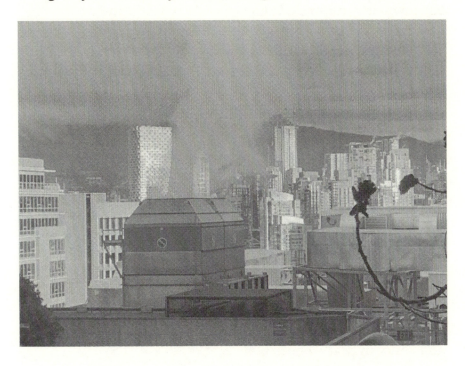

My golden view from the Seizures Investigations Unit, Vancouver General Hospital.

Sights and sounds from inside the SIU were unfamiliar and consumed calm. Seated with my laptop I was fully fenced in and alarm-guarded.

I used the remote to adjust the head of the bed frame to its highest position while I simultaneously ensured that the bed's movement hadn't affected the few electrical cords I'd plugged in. I didn't wanted them to be pinched or damaged. They were needed lifelines for communication, entertainment, and comfort.

What might the neurology team discover? Would I be

sentenced to life in bed without parole? The physical and cognitive decline I'd experienced in the last six months was devastating. Intense seizures appeared to have caused brain damage. I was reminded of Mom's failing brain and progressive dementia. Reminded that I was the one who'd placed her in care. She'd likely die there as a result. I didn't want to die here, and immediately stopped that train from proceeding down the track.

But, with increased frequency my thoughts climbed back on board and once again that train had started chugging. When would the whistle blow? And alarm, alert the SIU staff that I was seizing?

Right then, I made a conscious choice to see the bed I sat upon through a more hopeful lens. It wasn't helpful to gaze through a kaleidoscope of catastrophic fear.

I prayed God would provide what I so desperately needed through the hearts, hands, and gifted minds of highly skilled experts in their respective medical fields. Resolution was what I needed. Clarity and answers which would astound and convince this believer in her unbelief, that all would be well. And confirm that I would live.

~

I was appreciative to learn, after telling a nurse who'd dropped by that I was a hard target, that an IV specialty team was available, and would be called in.

It wasn't long until both the IV nurse and EEG technicians arrived. The first, to insert an access port, or intravenous line (IV), required to administer medication and fluids. The latter, to provide a miniscule amount of information about what to expect during their investigations. I did learn that I would be video-recorded twenty-four seven. And EEG technicians would consider my pulse and heartbeat, breathing, sweating, mouth, and muscle movements.

"Did you bring an electric toothbrush?" they asked. Various factors mimicked brain waves and thus could interfere and cause artifacts on an EEG recording. Apparently an electric toothbrush caused artifacts.

"Yes, I have one."

I was reminded to do anything I wanted, or needed to do, before the EEG team arrived to hook me up.

When an EEG technician returned, he glued electrodes, attached wires, and twisted, a funnel-like column of color-coded threads to my scalp. I affectionately called the braided, gauze-wrapped wires that tethered me to monitoring equipment my "brain umbilical cord," same as I had after my first EEG in February 2019. I'd tried to explain what it all looked like to Dale over the phone, and "brain umbilical cord" had suited the need for a descriptor, and stuck.

All wired up and plugged in, I was given a portable fabric fanny pack that could be slung over my shoulder, like those worn by bicycle couriers on city streets, which held the monitoring equipment temporarily, when required.

Getting out of bed was a big deal. A complicated procedure that required a call button, detaching wires, and the power source for my EEG equipment to be changed to battery operation. Alarms needed to be switched off, bed rails lowered, and that I shoulder the portable messenger's bag with the detached monitoring paraphernalia. I learned and understood. Leaving my bed was only to be done when absolutely required.

I closed my laptop and stored it temporarily where padded rails met bedding and considered a snack.

~

I hadn't decided which of the treats I brought from home, now stored in the top drawer of the rolling nightstand to eat, when I heard, "SEIZURE ALERT, SEIZURE ALERT, SEIZURE ALERT..."

An eardrum-piercing, eye-popping alarm loud enough to wake the dead demanded attention. And then, repeated:

"SEIZURE ALERT, SEIZURE ALERT, SEIZURE ALERT..."

Staff came running down the hallway towards my room, and just as I thought they'd enter, sequentially each turned left, and headed into the second of VGH's two-room, seizure unit.

~

I was told I could expect my evening meal tray to be delivered around five. But first I should expect various teams of specialists to visit. It was all part of the admissions protocol.

One after the other they arrived.

First, I met Dr. Hrazdil, pronounced "Razdil." She would take the neurology lead for the first two weeks, before Dr. Percy, my epileptologist, arrived for her fourteen-day neurology rotation at the SIU. Dr. Hrazdil would oversee my assessment and care. Next, there was a team from respirology for an initial consult to assess my history of shortness of breath, central apnea, and any correlation these might have to seizures.

I waited for the psychiatric team after the neurology and respiratory teams had come and gone. Cortisol flooded my nervous system, and I was in free fall. What if I learned that I had a life-shortening, degenerative diagnosis like Mom? I wasn't certain what to expect from either my body, or the neurological investigation.

Would what little faith I had be enough? Like when Peter walked on water towards Jesus, and believed he wouldn't sink? There was sure to be fierce storms and turbulent seas during my stay. Would God meet me in the turmoil and help me stay afloat? I needed to feel God's presence, know His firm grasp would keep and calm me and not let go. My thoughts shifted like a weather vane spinning and spiraling with uncertainty.

~

Questions stirred. Would the first seizure occur tonight while I slept, or need to be triggered? Would my mind and body under a microscope change its tune and be unable to provide sufficient evidence for claims I'd made? I had no idea. What I hadn't known, frightened me.

I needed to remind myself constantly, there could be *good news*, even if the burden of evidence to date appeared contradictory. I was in the care of a highly specialized team of experts.

*Be optimistic Jocelyn.*

My seizures had similarities and differences to those caused by epilepsy. I realized this after I read a booklet titled About Epilepsy months earlier at VGH's epilepsy clinic. I was hungry for understanding and a rotating rack offered a diverse selection of informational delicacies. I'd selected: Epilepsy —Seizures and First Aid, Epilepsy—A Guide for Teachers, and Epilepsy—A Guide for Professionals and Caregivers, and slipped the leaflets into my daypack. I hadn't known if I had epilepsy then but wanted to understand how to prepare if I did.

Information and facts calmed me. Facts provided certainty without lingering doubt. I needed certainty. An epileptic seizure, I learned, was a sudden, brief, and temporary disturbance of electrical activity in the brain. Often someone who suffers an epileptic seizure experiences a short period of unconsciousness. I hadn't been rendered lifeless or left in an unfeeling state by any of my seizures, nor had I lost bladder or bowel function at any time. These factors left my neurologists somewhat perplexed.

The neurology team listened then questioned to fill in any gaps in their understanding of what I'd experienced to date. Copious notes were taken. Dr. Hrazdil reiterated that I would be taken off seizure meds and allowed to use my CPAP for this first night only.

"Did I have any questions?" they asked.

I did, however I wasn't able to formulate any in a timely matter. The neurology team thanked me and left.

~

Epilepsy is one of the most common neurological conditions—an ancient disease, which has fascinated and frightened scientists; especially before there was a working knowledge of the central nervous system and seizures.

Would I be among the 1 percent of the global population, or the 65 million worldwide living with epilepsy?

*How could they be certain I didn't have it?*

A diagnosis would be considered if I had at least two unprovoked seizures occurring more than twenty-four hours apart, or one unprovoked seizure and appeared at risk of future unprovoked seizures.

As far as I could tell that made me an epileptic.

I had indefensible evidence of unprovoked seizures and that I was at risk for more. Dale and I could both provide expert testimony. People died prematurely from epilepsy, up to three times more frequently than the general population. I didn't want to be dead any time soon.

During medieval times pagans believed that seizures were a vengeance by the goddess of the moon. That the waxing moon supposedly heated the atmosphere surrounding the earth, which in turn melted the human's brain provoking seizures.

In the Middle Ages, when epilepsy was known as "the falling sickness," its victims were isolated from society, confined with the insane, and thought to be possessed by demons. Even their breath could infect an innocent bystander. I chuckled at the ridiculous notion that Dale could inhale my demonic spirits and experience seizures.

My distorted thoughts headed uphill on the world's tallest, longest, and fastest dive-coaster and were at the peak, just before the fall. I had that same visceral sensation as I sat tethered, waiting to seize.

~

Last to arrive was Dr. Sidhu, for an initial psychiatric consultation. Dr. Percy reiterated that I would be assessed by various specialties, however I wasn't prepared for a psychiatrist to be accompanied by extra listeners. The few experiences I had to date with psychiatric assessment were with a single practitioner in a private setting.

Each specialist in the seizure unit brought fellows, postgraduate medical trainees undertaking post-certification specialty training. VGH is a teaching hospital that partners with the University of British Columbia, a global centre for research and teaching.

Dr. Sidhu was the first to speak.

"Hello Jocelyn, I'm Dr. Sidhu." I tried to focus my attention and listening solely on Dr. Sidhu, so as not to be overwhelmed. Others standing around the peripheral of the room became invisible. He hadn't started out asking, "How are you?" Instead, he'd smiled and offered, "It's lovely to meet you, Jocelyn." I was able to offer a genuine smile as I exhaled, and my shoulders relaxed, a little.

He'd invested in the relationship and simultaneously created a reassuring space.

"How can I help you?" he asked, then waited patiently. I sensed he wasn't in a hurry and that I wasn't just another patient.

I gathered my thoughts, considered where to start, and vented.

First impressions matter. My initial impression was that Dr. Sidhu saw me as smart and capable of making healthy choices and decisions about my care. I'd needed that.

He took the time, gently encouraged, and honoured my intelligence. He invited me to believe he would be fully invested in my care. He hadn't interrupted my words or thoughts as they stampeded out.

Relief flooded my emotionally triggered brain as Dr. Sidhu listened. I was over-tired and allowed tears to fall when they came. He created a brave space that enabled me to experience being authentically heard for the first time. He hadn't made assumptions, arrived with preconceived judgement, accused, or shamed me.

With a smile and nonjudgmental body language he offered an invitation to proceed slowly and safely at my own pace. I sensed I could trust, tell the truth, and would be believed.

I authentically expressed my feelings. I shared from my depths for only the second time. The first was when I told Dale I loved him, in 1982. I don't let down my guard easily.

I turned to Dr. Sidhu and realized I could trust him. There wasn't a need to shield myself or dole out intellectual bullshit to mask my pain, as I had with so many others.

I started by telling him how I felt about "D-Day," January 27, 2020. A day when I lost so much of what mattered: my newly earned role as a teacher-librarian, driver's licence, and independence. On a roll, I travelled back in time. I explained the loss of my sacred safe space when Mom moved into our home, that her dementia journey became front and center and I her full-time care-partner and power of attorney, and the torment and decision to place Mom in care, which had fallen to me.

Without taking a breather or pause to exhale, tears fell as I told Dr. Sidhu about my physical and cognitive decline. I peeled back the layers, one at a time.

Pain oozed from my core and leaked from cells where my body had locked away traumatic memories. Incidents that I'd been unable to grieve. Incidents that had shamed. Events when malicious words were spewed, had wounded, and caused irreparable damage.

Through tears, I explained unresolved grief I'd needed to store when it wasn't safe to respond, react, or use my voice.

"How can I help?" Dr. Sidhu said. He already had. Dr. Sidhu witnessed my story and believed me. He witnessed unresolved grief carried since toddlerhood—grief that still lingered more than fifty years later.

I was and am an intelligent, capable educational leader. I was and am highly professional. I'd been deeply wounded, and my voice taken. Dr. Sidhu created the necessary conditions which enabled me to find my voice and trust that I could use it. He gifted his presence, his expertise, and cared enough to listen.

Dr. Sidhu tuned in and gave an audience to my grief. Verbal diarrhea flooded the room as I spoke of a biological father who'd abandoned his parenting responsibility.

"I was only two."

Mom, I explained, did everything within her power to give us a wonderful life. The life she wanted for us and perhaps hadn't had.

Were there good-night kisses? I couldn't remember.

~

I hadn't had a parent to turn to at four, fourteen, twenty-four, or fifty-four when I was in pain, and hadn't wanted to burden my mother, or husband. Would he understand? I hadn't wanted to give him any reason to leave.

There'd been a dear friend killed in a freak accident. Why had a horse been accidentally loose and roaming on the highway in the dark? There was a near-death kayaking mishap in my twenties about which I hadn't trusted anyone with the knowledge of that terror. Through each successive decade I struggled to articulate my fears.

I was overjoyed in my thirties to have had the opportunity to choose to be a stay-at-home mom, with Dale's full support. However, when I attempted to return to teaching, I'd needed the thickened skin of a rhinoceros to manage my emotions. I had twelve job interviews in a single year, only to be told, "We'd love to hire you, Jocelyn, and it's evident that you are an exceptional candidate." But always someone else secured the job.

Had they already had someone in mind? It seemed that way. Repeated layoffs year after year through my late thirties and forties wreaked havoc.

The unexpected landslide beneath my feet at fifty broke me.

Each loss alone was significant. Together, the sum was too much. Without resilience or skills for supporting emotional regulation or distress tolerance, a parent or mentor to provide empathy or compassion, I stood on a precipice.

Standing on that ledge, I hadn't wanted to die, although traumatic incidents stored as memories in my body's physiology needed to be discharged. My body had tallied and kept the score.

~

Since the 1900s phenobarbital and the Keto diet were used to manage epilepsy before the evolution of modern antiepileptic drugs. Both of my AEDs, topiramate and Brivlera, were prescribed to prevent first myoclonic jerks, then seizures.

I'd needed the seizure meds. That's why they were prescribed. Dale reassured me he believed that they made a difference. I'd thought so, too, but I trusted Dale's judgement most, knowing my own cognition was poor and in decline.

I wanted to be calm on Day One at the SIU, but seizures had occurred daily. Would they escalate in frequency, intensity, and duration now that I was no longer medicated with AEDs?

Truth be told, I was scared.

~

I attempted sleep that first night and, not unexpectedly, had a seizure.

"SEIZURE ALERT, SEIZURE ALERT, SEIZURE ALERT!"

The seizure didn't last long, but staff came running straight towards my room without turning left. As my body rocked and convulsed, they stripped away blankets to observe and allow cameras to record. All the while asking questions.

"What's this? And this?" One of the nurses had the responsibility of selecting items one at a time, holding each up in front of my face, encouraging me to speak, identify small objects, and follow simple instructions as I seized.

I'd noticed the bin filled with an odd assortment earlier on the window ledge as I unpacked, but hadn't known what they were for.

"Point to the wall with the window." Then, "What day of the week is today?" "Tell me where you are?" She peppered me with these, and other equally challenging questions while I hoped the seizure would stop. Her inquiries continued till the seizure ended, and even then didn't stop. I sighed deeply, closed my eyes, and prayed I'd be able to sleep. But rest wasn't an option as the questions continued.

Another of the nurses reminded me of a request previously made that I'd forgotten in the chaos as I seized.

She pointed to one of two push-buttons at my bedside placed expressly to be within reach when required.

"If you think you're going to experience another seizure, please be sure to press the button." Then added, only after I'd opened my eyes, "This red one." She continued to point, hoping my flickering lids would reopen long enough to acknowledge her request. She pressed on until weary pupils were drawn toward her pointing finger and correctly identified the red button.

I'd remembered that I was supposed to do *something* but hadn't remembered what. When I did remember and reached in the confusion (*Was it this one?*), my fingers had become talons, my head rotated without reason, and fearful eyes scanned.

I was not in control or able to push the RED, or any other button.

I couldn't answer the nurse's questions initially. My jaw was clamped shut. I couldn't verbalize though I'd recognized a comb, a pencil case, and the plastic replica of a striped carnivorous feline that the nurse held up...

"T-Tiger?" It hadn't appeared to matter if I was right. She'd dropped the tiger back into the bin and pulled out a plastic utensil.

"Spoon," I answered with clarity, then remembered I'd borrowed this exact spoon from the blue plastic tote she now held when I'd wanted to eat a container of tapioca pudding I'd brought from home. There'd been no other cutlery in sight. Had they recorded the look of disgust on my face when it occurred to me how many different hands must have touched THAT SPOON prior to me naming it?

Seizure #1 was now recorded history. Reassured, I hoped for sleep.

~

I awakened periodically throughout the night, just

like when I was away camping or staying at a hotel in an unfamiliar bed. I heard beeping, ticking, traffic and wailing sirens, as ambulances arrived to VGH's emergency department. Lights streamed into the room through the curtained entry and, without a closed door, made escaping distractions and finding sleep near impossible.

It was understandable that closed doors and darkened hospital rooms weren't practical where life support might be required without warning. But the semi-opaque fabric-panelled curtain parading as a door enabled bright light to stream above, below, and through it. This made reaching REM, the deepest stage of sleep, beyond the bounds of possibility.

As promised, I was permitted my CPAP machine that first night but told I would not be allowed it on subsequent nights. The following morning a nurse returned, and I needed to make an extremely difficult decision.

"Which six hours would you like to sleep tonight?" asked the nurse at seven in the morning. "The doctor has giving instructions to recreate conditions which will trigger seizures. We'll be starting a sleep deprivation schedule tonight."

Admitted less than twenty-four hours, I'd already experienced a couple of small seizures and little sleep. The nurse stood brows raised awaiting my answer. I chose midnight to 6 a.m. Drained of energy, fatigued by interrupted rest, I needed to keep myself awake for the next seventeen hours.

I struggled to fill the endless hours when I wasn't supposed to sleep and listened through the hospital room's headwall where electrical and medical gas outlets were. It became apparent that the walls weren't completely soundproofed. I listened intently to conversations which were sometimes muffled and on occasion crystal clear.

I was pretty sure that on the other side of the wall EEG technicians huddled around their equipment and monitors in a room that doubled as a space for specialists to collaborate. My intellectual curiosity was piqued. I loved that I could hear specialists strategizing and discussing the infamous "abnormal" discharges: mine.

Knowing that a think tank of experts was convened on the other side of the wall made me feel tethered and secure one minute and terrified the next.

My days were a blur of exhaustion, with brief interruptions as I seized. *Brief,* as if "brief" was defined as seemingly never-ending, despite of a short duration.

Thoughts invaded, and I catastrophized, worried, prayed, remembered the terror of the last dizzying loop and coaster car in free fall. Then I hit the curve and, exhausted, dozed. Exhaustion triggered seizures, and I'd seize, think, worry, pray and circle back for another loop on the coaster from hell… repeated ad nauseum.

I needed to get off this terrifying ride, buckled in, as I was for the duration.

~

I needed a lift. After all, it was Valentine's Day. I changed out of my pajama top and buttoned up a cherry-red, buttery soft blouse with decorative floral embroidery. It made me feel appropriately dressed for a celebration of romance.

I am a huge fan of silky textures that caress my skin, and not so much an aficionada of the cylindrical weave of colour-coded wires attached to my scalp. I waited for a prearranged video call with My Valentine. My gauze-wrapped weave didn't complement the look I was going for, but Dale wouldn't mind.

Nobody cared in 2020-21, on Zoom or any other video conferencing platform, what was worn below the waist. I completed my eye-catching look with blue and white polka-dotted, fleece pajama pants. Then sent a rouge Dior lipstick-kiss emoji to Dale letting him know I was dressed and ready for our Valentine's Day date.

As expected, my phone rang.

"How's my Valentine?" Dale inquired.

*Better now.* "Happy Valentine's Day," I replied with a smile. "I'm wishing you were here."

"You know I want to be."

"You'll never guess what I got for breakfast today," I said.

I didn't want to start our date with a seizure report, or tell Dale I was panic-stricken, or paralyzed with fear while I seized in the night. Those hadn't seemed great Valentine's Day conversation starters and would likely kill the mood.

I knew Dale would be concerned for me due to his lack of proximity. Not by choice, but because of mandated pandemic necessity. I chose instead to share an anecdote. Earlier in the day I'd laughed out loud, a true belly laugh. Momentarily, the incident created calm, and I was able to temporarily escape the coaster from hell.

Now I was giddy, a kid telling a joke with my dimples on display. I turned my laptop's camera. Filling the screen was my tray and a circular pre-warmed plate with an insulated green plastic lid ensuring it hadn't arrived cold. Opening the lid, I exclaimed, "Voila! One, freshly-cooked, hard-boiled egg, and... NOTHING else."

I have a weird sense of humour and was the only one laughing. Dale smiled and with raised brows emitted a composed, three-syllable chuckle: "Mmm." It was a silly moment but felt perfect.

~

Shortly after breakfast EEG technicians returned. While one checked and reglued electrodes to ensure correct positioning of each, the other explained that something had interfered with yesterday's recordings during my seizure. Technicians were baffled as to the cause and searched all around the bed and hospital's head wall system behind me where electrical and medical gas functions were organized to ensure a safe productive space, especially in the event of an emergency.

After they completed a meticulous search, they'd come across my extension cord. "What have you got plugged into this extension cord?"

"My cell phone and laptop chargers," I replied.

"Those shouldn't have affected our recordings or caused an artifact." The way they spoke, it was apparent they were thinking out loud. It wasn't about me.

"Have you got anything else plugged in?"

It took me a few moments to visualize, and then it came to me. I'd forgotten to tell them about my electric heating pad. I hadn't thought anything more of it, after I'd arranged and tucked it beneath the covers. Indeed, it was the problematic artifact.

I was sad to lose a valued creature comfort which provided pain relief and warmth to frequently chilled extremities. I reluctantly conceded that what I deemed essential, was in fact not. I wrapped the cord around the blanket to be put away. I felt bad. It must have caused technicians, as well as specialists, unnecessary shoulder shrugging, increased blood pressure, and unwanted stress.

A rubber band snapped and there'd been another seizure. Sudden seizures followed periods of calm and caused my reptilian brain to freeze.

Afterward I wondered, how much more of this can I take? What if they don't learn what causes my seizures?

~

I hadn't believed I was smart. In fact, I couldn't remember every believing it. I competed for affection, compared myself to others, and found myself lacking. I learned to bottle my feelings, manage what I could, and hoped no one would find out that I wasn't as capable as I tried so hard to appear. I observed a parent and learned that anger and fighting weren't acceptable for good girls. *Perhaps, if I was good, I'd be loveable*, I thought.

~

I estimated the hourly cost of my care each day, as specialists and technicians collaborated. My brain doesn't shut down easily or often. I've always been a curious kid—now in a less than perfect body, getting older year after year, but no less curious.

I was grateful that at the end of what might be a twenty-one-day stay multiplied by the cost of care provided wouldn't be a sum I would be responsible to pay. Unlike our neighbours to the south, in the USA. I was relieved to know that in British Columbia, Medical Services Plan (MSP) premiums were eliminated January 1, 2020, and I was able to concentrate on getting better, rather than how Dale and I would afford what otherwise would undoubtedly be crippling debt.

~

"Tonight, you may have four hours of permitted sleep," the nurse said. "Would you prefer to sleep between midnight and 0400, or between 0200-0600?"

Surely, she was kidding, I hoped. Her tone suggested otherwise.

With a total of six hours of sleep since I'd arrived at VGH I realized afterward that this meant staying awake through the day, past midnight, and until 2 a.m. I wasn't sure I could. In fact, I was certain I couldn't.

"Can I have an afternoon nap?"

With the inner corners of her brows raised, and lips pulled down, she shook her head and left me with, "Sorry, no."

~

Dr. Sidhu dropped by Tuesday night and told me about UBC's neuropsychiatry program. He felt I would be well suited. "I'd love to see you get into the program, Jocelyn." Then he added, "I can get to work tonight on a referral if you think you'd be interested."

I was desperate for support and extremely keen. If Dr. Sidhu believed this was what I needed, I wanted it.

The muscles around his eyes tightened, his cheeks lifted, and his lips parted as he thanked me with a genuine smile. "Thank you for your courage and time, Jocelyn."

~

"Good night, my handsome Swede. I love you."

I clicked the red stop sign and *ended* our Tuesday evening, late night check-in after Dr. Sidhu was on his way.

Dale had reassured me that he would be arriving in Vancouver Friday afternoon. I couldn't wait to wrap my arms around the love of my life and be the recipient of one of his soul-reviving hugs.

More than once I needed to shake off sleep. I watched thrillers; drank fluids, which created a requirement that I get up and out of bed; and watched the clock. After the dinner tray was taken at 1900 hour and before 2100 arrived was the most difficult. I seriously considered phoning a friend or requesting someone to sit with me. It was a tortuous endeavor to stay awake, as I watched the clock mesmerized by the silent tick, tick, ticking of the second hand as it made its way painfully around the circumference of the clock.

I waited for midnight long after binging Netflix could successfully keep my lids from drooping. I experienced sudden, brief, and strong contractions in my head and neck as my brain-case repeatedly drooped and my body expressed that sleep was a prerequisite for continued function.

Where there's a will, I found a way. I wouldn't allow myself to fall asleep as a matter of principle. I was obsessive in my need to demonstrate that I had what it took. I could demonstrate the required self-control, I reminded myself, hearing Kristen repeat what she'd told me earlier when she'd come to visit: "You've got this, Mom." I was a rule follower and using a less complimentary expression, legalistically black and white in my thinking. At 0200, I'd have either demonstrated I could do it or would be the world's biggest failure.

I listened to obnoxious, eardrum-impairing tunes on Spotify. Not by choice, but out of necessity. I snacked and considered phoning folks I didn't like. And eventually, even those I loved, but hated at this hour knowing they were sleeping soundly. It wasn't fair.

I wondered, as I tried to stay awake, if I truly needed to accept my current physical health and cognitive decline. *Could I?*

I couldn't. I would not! I could not get used to the idea

that at fifty-seven it would all be downhill. It wouldn't be if I had any say; except I didn't seem to have any say in the matter. Perhaps if I looked through a pair of rose-coloured sunglasses.

~

It hadn't taken long to forget that I'd surrendered mid-January to a higher power and vowed to trust. In the wee hours after midnight Tuesday, when employees on the graveyard shift at the hospital were freshly showered and energetic, I prayed.

> *Dearest Lord Jesus,*
> *You are not a far off, impersonal god unconcerned and unfamiliar with my seasons of suffering, or the worries of my daily life. Thank you for being a savior that cares about my physical and spiritual condition. Give me a spirit of humility as I rely on your Holy Spirit to cultivate hope within me. May this hope result in praise and honor to you, and a desire to share this hope with others. As I await your return, may I continue to put my hope in you, following you faithfully no matter my earthly circumstances.*
> *I surrender... I'm not in control! Amen.*

~

Dried glue that secured electrodes to my scalp caused a burning sensation and irritating itch. Painful cracks had developed in the specialized adhesive, I later learned was called collodion, and I needed the equivalent of a thick moisturizer with a skin-softening agent. Not for dry skin, but for my scalp in each location where electrodes were anchored. Could I wait another fifty-eight hours for a shower? I hadn't wanted to imagine another sixteen days at the SIU, but I easily could.

I was ready to attempt sleep and finally allowed to rest, but my busy brain had other ideas as I contemplated the silliness of counting sheep and waited for a psyche-invigorating, bear hug from Dale.

Only three more sleeps. Then, perhaps I'd escape this

solitary confinement and tormented tunnel of worry and be in Dale's arms.

In our late twenties, Dale and I, and our dear friends Ken and Jill, climbed down into an underground labyrinth through a subway-sized tunnel that plunged steeply. We'd planned for a sunny day of boating, but grey skies and a light rain dampened our enthusiasm. We'd decided to go spelunking instead.

We'd moved to the remote west coast village of Tahsis, in 1991, and were told by a local that Coral Cave was just up the logging road west from the turnaround at West Bay. A short trail would lead us to the cave's entrance."

We successfully found the entrance, geared up, and headed in and down. We didn't realize that a sprinkle would become a downpour, or that puddles that threatened dry socks through waterproof boots would become knee-deep plunge pools. I definitely didn't anticipate a river to funnel over ledges we'd cautiously descended with a force that both hindered and hastened our escape.

One moment we were joyfully exploring. The next, we were fleeing like prehistoric reptiles at the end of the Mesozoic Era, 65 million years ago, and desperate to witness a tell-tale spark of light that would register and convey we'd live another day.

I was elevated and experienced manic urgency in 1991, and each time a seizure struck thirty years later.

Still in bed, it was the fifth of what Dr. Percy had indicated might be a twenty-one-day caving expedition. I finally seized the opportunity and slumbered.

JOCELYN BYSTROM

# CHAPTER TWENTY-TWO

## FiNDing Hope

Early Wednesday morning, to my complete surprise, the neurology team reassembled. Three neurologists filed into my room and spread themselves, at equal intervals, around my bed in a semicircle. Later I realized they'd most likely been social distancing due to mandated pandemic protocols. I hadn't put two and two together at the time.

Dr. Hradzil greeted me warmly and gave Dr. Nedd a nod.

Dr. Nedd had been present most days and checked in with me often. She arrived with what I suspected were diagnostic hypotheses and questioned me to ensure she hadn't erroneously missed any indispensable detail. A thorough, collaborative care physician, she provided compassionate care, like Dr. Sidhu, and returned to give me updates and information I'd hoped to hear.

"I thought you might like to be kept up to date about what we're seeing," she said.

She was correct. I required updates to discharge fear and appreciated her intuition. She was able to read me easily after our first meeting. She observed facial expressions, non-verbal body language, and listened too. One evening she arrived later than expected, and after she'd already visited earlier that same day. It was apparent she'd worked longer than a twelve-hour shift.

"Have you eaten your dinner yet?" I'd inquired.

I wasn't surprised by her answer. I encouraged her to head home, saying, "You've got to look after yourself, rest, and recharge. I'll still be here in the morning."

She was young and keen, and I presumed an overachiever. It was apparent she cared deeply about her life's work and the patients in her care. I saw her, I knew the type. I was like that. I *am* like that, except no longer young, or a neurology fellow, like Dr. Nedd.

Now, observing my nod, Dr. Nedd began to report what the neurology team had learned to date.

"Before you share any news," I interrupted, "can we wait till I call Dale on my phone to join us, please?

I wanted to be able to remember what they said and wouldn't unless Dale was able to listen and record. I needed Dale to remind me later of the specifics, after I may have forgotten or not coded.

Drs. Hrazdil and Nedd simultaneously chuckled.

"Of course!"

I retrieved my cell phone from the over-bed table and dialed. Would Dale be available on a weekday morning? It was typically his busiest time of day. He might be out on a jobsite or driving. He wouldn't be expecting a call.

He answered after just a few rings.

"Hi Hon," I said. "I'm here in my room with the neurology team. They want to share their findings to date. Are you able to take the time, right now, to listen and take notes?"

"Absolutely!" They gave him time to "teleport" into the room and get his mind recalibrated for what lay ahead. They keenly assumed that he'd want to record any diagnostic information and care instructions in his notebook. Another accurate assumption.

Dale's my person.

"I'm ready, thanks for your patience," Dale chimed in.

Dr. Nedd continued. "We've just arrived and are able to tell you both that we have the best news ever." She paused briefly, not for dramatic effect, but to draw breath and continue.

"We usually have to tell patients they've been diagnosed with epilepsy, and share difficult news with our patients and their loved ones."

With my headed angled toward Dr. Nedd, like our cocker spaniel Ollie's when he's curious, I concentrated with profound intensity. I monitored every syllable, nuance, and expression Dr. Nedd emitted, and imagined Dale was as well.

"Today, we're able to tell you both that a diverse group of experts have read and reviewed Jocelyn's numerous EEG scans, those recorded between 2013–2021, in addition to those we've observed here in the seizure unit. We were fortunate and able to record ten seizures in just five days. We've been able to collaborate and determine after extensive discussion that there's nothing neurologically wrong with Jocelyn's brain."

Dr. Nedd paused, then reiterated what she'd said moments earlier, perhaps to let the significance of the findings sink in.

"This is the best news that we ever get to give, and don't get to share often." Recognition dawned and pursed lips I'd imagined, after countless hours of wide-eyed concentration and half-lidded investigation, now sparkled as smile lines eased across their faces.

I sat stunned and didn't understand. It must have been apparent to everyone as they'd read my facial expression. I wondered what Dale was thinking.

"The epileptic-appearing discharges which first appeared on Jocelyn's EEG scans in 2013, were marked as abnormal," Dr. Nedd continued. "When in fact they'd been correctly identified by one of Jocelyn's neurologists, after a second EEG, with sleep deprivation, as normal."

*Wait, what?* I was completely flummoxed.

"Why, then have I been experiencing exponentially

increasing seizures and cognitive decline?" It didn't add up.

Dr. Nedd elaborated in the hope that I'd understand.

"Experts were called in from retirement and extensive research was completed. An extensive team of specialists across varied neurology disciplines pulled out every stop. We even pulled out and reviewed old, outdated textbooks. Neurologists from across North America have read and consulted on Jocelyn's scans."

After a short hesitation as if to collect her thoughts, Dr. Nedd detailed what they could now confidently confirm.

"What we're seeing is extremely rare. Jocelyn..." She waited till my eyes met hers. "Your discharges, which continue to appear on your scans, and have since 2013, are a very rare normal variant." I wondered if Dale was chuckling.

*He apparently proposed to a very rare, odd duck.*

Dr. Nedd paused, ready to reiterate and embellish if I still didn't *get it*. The feeling of being overwhelmed must have been painted on my face, as Dr. Nedd appeared to be completing-a full-body scan in search for clues. Had she noted the tilt of my head, me scratching my face, and the positioning of my brows?

Her smiling eyes and dimples aimed to ensure I was reassured. Just in case I wasn't, she restated the diagnosis once again:

"Your discharges have been reclassified by a highly specialized team of scholars and recategorized as a very rare, normal variant."

She stopped periodically, as if to wait for my dense neural circuitry to catch up and respond. Dr. Nedd paused to give 100 billion neurons—with 100 trillion connections—an opportunity to send mixed messages in the hope that I'd receive corrected information.

"There's nothing ... neurologically ... wrong with your brain."

I sat stupefied as I considered Dale seated and listening to this news in his work truck. He was probably all business and no fear. He's calm in the eye of a storm. His cell phone would be microphone up in his left chest pocket, enabling him to hear, speak, and have hands free to record what we were hearing.

The neurology team might have skipped buoyantly from the room they were so pleased. But Dr. Nedd's comedic punchline was still to come. With a wide grin she thought to raise my spirits one more notch.

"You'll be able to drive again."

There was a long-protracted silence.

I burst into maniacal laughter. *No way was I going to be driving any time soon.* Dale, listening on the phone, I was certain concurred.

*That's crazy!* Beyond crazy; that's irrational. Allowing someone who's just experienced ten seizures in the last five days to drive was insane. I must have misheard. Had she said I could drive?

She had.

Realizing that what she'd just announced was meant to be obviously comprehended as in six months to a year's time, Dr. Nedd wisely backtracked.

"Not right away, of course." I couldn't believe it. Seconds earlier, I'd believed I would never again turn a key in an ignition.

Dr. Hrazdil summarized.

The new diagnosis: functional neurologic disorder, or FND, was explained in less words than a typical tweet.

"It's a disorder in the realm of neuropsychology."

"Neuropsychology?" *What on earth was that?* Psychology, I knew, was the study of the human mind, but neuropsychology? Would a neuropsychologist be able to stop the onset of seizures? I couldn't conjure how.

Drs. Hrazdil and Nedd didn't arrogantly pretend to be exceptionally knowledgeable about FND. I took this to mean that functional neurologic disorder was somewhat outside the realm of neurology. Whose specialty, if not neurology?

What I hadn't known then was that a neuropsychologist studies how a person's cognition and behaviour are related to the brain and nervous system. Neurologists and psychiatrists both work to treat diseases that affect the brain and mind. Neurologists, like Drs. Hrazdil and Percy, specialized in the science related to epilepsy.

Neurologists specialize in physiological illnesses, or physical health. While psychiatrists, like Dr. Sidhu, specialized in psychological disorders.

It would have been good to have had help understanding these distinctions as I frantically attempted to sort this all out while seated in the SIU after unexpectedly hearing I had FND.

I needed a few signposts along the way.

For seven years I was advocating for physical care in all the wrong places. How many others were like me? Where were all the signs along the way that ought to have pointed me in a different direction? I'd left the realm of neurology and physical health and entered the domain of mental health. That was certainly something surprising to wrap my head around.

*Did I have a mental illness that caused seizures?*

Next, my neurologists suggested a workbook. How was a *workbook* going to help resolve prevalent and disabling seizures? The title of the workbook though piqued my interest: *Taking Control of Your Seizures: Treatments That Work.*

I guessed it could be worth a try.

My seizures were lions and wouldn't be easily tamed or domesticated. They had an aggressive instinct for the wild. Each terrifying event robbed me of self-control. It was most definitely not going to be easy to turn that around. I couldn't imagine using my wits to disarm the beast. Wasn't that the role of someone who'd successfully attempted to expel or drive out demons?

I needed Jesus, not an exorcist.

"Once you get home you can read and review

information about FND and order the workbook," they suggested. They also highly recommended two websites—neurosymptoms.org and FNDhope.org—to assist us in understanding my new and unexpected FND diagnosis.

Wait until I got home? *They had to be kidding.* As soon as their lab coattails exited the room, I opened my laptop and fled to find hope.

Seizures, although a significant worry as I mentally prepared to be discharged, weren't my only concern. What about my impaired cognition and inability to code information during what had now been reclassified as "very rare normal" discharges.

Just because they'd been named "NORMAL" didn't mean my cognition was. A thick medical record, which included extensive cognitive testing results completed before Christmas, 2020 testified to that. I didn't get it.

My doctors, not skilled at mind reading, hadn't answered when I peppered them with questions posed as thoughts. I wasn't afraid to ask, I just hadn't.

Dr. Nedd suggested that after I arrived home and while I waited for Dr Sidhu to complete the referral to UBC's neuropsychiatry program, a referral they'd known he was working on, that I might want to locate a counsellor locally in the Comox Valley. Perhaps they believed it would be simple to find a neuropsychologist who was FND aware conducting therapy via a video-conferencing platform during a global pandemic, who'd be familiar and willing to guide me through the specific seizures investigation workbook they'd recommended. It was not!

There was a shortage of neuropsychologists across the province doing therapeutic work with patients. Most who were, weren't taking on new clients. Perhaps I could try to locate a therapist or counsellor able to facilitate the lessons designed to be completed collaboratively with a trained therapist.

"It might be tough, but we'll keep looking for

a neuropsychiatrist on your behalf," Dr. Nedd reassured. "Though it might not be right away. Most have capped their waiting lists."

I wasn't interested in waiting. I went online and promptly purchased both the workbook and therapist's guide. I can be impulsive in that way when it comes to managing fear. I wanted to have the books ready and in hand when I found someone adequately prepared AND willing to make sense of *my very rare normal brain.*

I'd pass them the therapist's guide saying, "Let's get started."

~

My mind flooded with questions. Not the least of which was how to manage seizures without medication. What was the plan if I continued to have as many seizures in the next five days as I had in the last?

I was to be discharged from Vancouver General's SIU first thing the following morning. What about Thursday, Friday, and Saturday? Never mind the days, weeks, and months ahead.

I tried to be grateful for the emotional release after learning that I didn't have a brain tumor, cancer, multiple sclerosis, Parkinson's, or epilepsy. *But what about the seizures?*

In all my reading and research in the last seven years, as I'd anxiously fretted about what was wrong with me, I'd never run into articles or research about FND.

I'm functional . . . but disordered? I had a fierce determination to create my own plan since the doctors hadn't said anything about a referral to an FND specialist. Certainly, there had to be someone who'd completed their doctoral dissertation on functional neurological disorder, who could help me make sense of it all.

I didn't cry; I wasn't sad. There was no great epiphany after my FND diagnosis. Why hadn't specialists mentioned the possibility of this diagnosis sooner? My mind flooded with questions. Why had neurologists spent all this time, expense, and investigation, only to tell me that I could head to the

World Wide Web and figure things out for myself. My curious and intelligent brain devoured information about FND that late afternoon, as I sat on my discharge-bed reading and researching to learn what the heck it meant to have FND.

Young people, I discovered, experienced a unique set of challenges during the COVID-19 pandemic, and it was widely reported that for one in five there would be a negative impact on their mental health. Could they get FND? Would they experience unexpected functional symptoms in the years ahead? I hoped not.

Who would decide after copious data was collected what funding was required for the repercussions of the pandemic on our children, and youth? These will be the next generations' leaders, politicians, and decision-makers.

I'm just one individual with FND. *Anyone* could develop it, I read. An estimated one per ten thousand population worldwide may experience functional symptoms, or eventually be diagnosed with FND. That number seemed highly undercounted.

Doctors have been investigating me for seven years and they just now realized I have FND. There must be a significant number of individuals suffering in silence without required supports or FND aware medical practitioners. What of the youth of tomorrow who may not have the required mental health support or medical practitioners who are yet unaware that traumatic incidents experienced during a global pandemic may take a decade to show up?

The Comox Valley had a population of 72,500 in 2021, and our North Island Hospital's- Comox Valley Campus location doesn't have a neurology department. No one I know of knew about FND previously or its connection to the seizures I experienced. The numbers of individuals struggling to manage functional symptoms without adequate supports must be exponential.

At FNDhope.org, I read that "despite the prevalence of functional neurological disorder, exact causes are unknown."

Another research report indicated approximately one-third of neurology outpatients reported functional symptoms, and that many different predisposing factors make patients susceptible. Head injuries (i.e., concussions), auto-accidents, back injuries, surgeries (post-operative), and even non-physical stressful events. Some FND diagnosed individuals reported they had no predisposing factors whatsoever.

Throughout my diagnostic journey I sensed an impairment of my self-agency. I wasn't in control of the functional symptoms I experienced: migraines, myoclonic jerks, seizures, and/or cognitive decline. Nor had I done anything to cause them.

Psychological and traumatic life events may be risk factors for developing FND, but rarely provide a full explanation for the underlying causes. Diagnosed individuals aren't necessarily stressed, depressed, or anxious when they develop functional symptoms. They may not have had adverse childhood experiences, I learned.

The lack of easy-to-understand facts available after an FND diagnosis left me reading well past sunset and kept me awake even later than when I'd been on a regimental sleep schedule limiting my sleep. I binged online rather than on Netflix to find FND facts. I viewed informative videos until long after it had all become a monotone cocktail of blah blah blah.

"Blah blah blah… something about having experienced trauma… blah blah blah…there are predisposing factors."

~

The respiratory team crossed the threshold into my room a short while later. I'd barely had time to learn the basics about FND online. They'd reviewed their findings and found nothing unexpected. Yes, I had asthma. Yes, my known allergies could have easily triggered and contributed to challenged breathing. Yes, laboured breathing and anxiety may have brought on functional symptoms. No surprises, no enlightenment.

No new medications were required or prescribed. Their final analysis—I would be re-referred for a two-day overnight sleep assessment at the UBC Sleep Disorders Clinic. I hoped this second referral would prompt action sooner than my first had.

I hadn't remembered to request Dale listen or record what the respirology team shared. Had my subconscious known Dale needed to get back to work, and that there'd be another more important call?

~

There wasn't much of an interval and the nurse arrived to tell me that Dr. Sidhu's team would be in shortly.

"Call me as soon as Dr. Sidhu's team arrives," Dale had reminded me. We both sensed this his might be more informative. He knew I would call, and I knew he'd be waiting. We'd hung up without debriefing after the neurology team's report. We were both abundantly clear what "shortly" meant.

We had no words. Our minds were overfull.

~

Meanwhile, I sat gobsmacked. How could there be nothing neurologically wrong with me? I'd just had ten seizures in short order. There'd be no new meds and in fact the neurology team recommended I discontinue all antiepileptics medications. I believed that prescribed drugs I'd been taking up until February 12, 2021, were working and reduced the frequency, intensity, and duration of daily seizures.

*What now?*

Good news usually ruptures hopelessness, changes dispositions with hope, and brings joy to the darkest hours. How could it be considered good news to be told I was going home with no proactive plan to reduce seizures? Their description of "THE BEST NEWS EVER" terrified me!

~

I dialed Dale's cell when I heard Dr. Sidhu outside my door speaking with Dr. Nedd. When his team returned, we were ready.

Dr. Hrazdil's team sparked hope. I prayed Dr. Sidhu's

team would fan the flame the neurologists kindled, and with less spine-chilling, good news.

In a manner I'd come to appreciate, Dr. Sidhu got straight to the point. Dr. Sidhu listened without interrupting. He arrived with a cell phone on his hip and an imaginary black leather doctor's bag. In it I believed were significant expertise, abundant professionalism, the wisdom of King Solomon, and perhaps a defunct lab coat. He hadn't needed to carry a copy of the text that I thought ought to be prescribed for every medical student, *The Physicians Book of Etiquette & Manual of Politeness*. Dr. Sidhu already personified what every health care consumer hoped for from their medical doctor.

With Dale listening, he began.

"I finished filling out your referral to UBC's neuropsychiatry program and I sincerely hope you get in. It may be difficult as their intake has an extensive waitlist. However, I believe you would respond extremely well to treatment. In the interim I've also contacted Comox Valley Mental Health with a referral for you to a local psychiatrist there. They'll be able to provide some support to get you started."

I was laser focused on his words, wanting to hear and understand the forward-thinking treatment plan, which I hoped would reassure my disquieted spirit. My brain seemed stuck, stalled, and frozen as I'd watched Dr. Sidhu's mouth become a source of sounds and speech filling a container. Mine had already overflowed.

I hoped Dale was recording. I caught snippets. Dr. Sidhu pulled me back to the present as I'd heard my name.

"Jocelyn, your FND diagnosis triple-checks all the required boxes."

Dr. Sidhu paused. Had he observed immobilized eyes and a frozen demeanor? What were the tells that caused him to pause? Had he witnessed confusion or was it his finely-tuned acuity that'd enabled him to comprehend, and know, I'd fled the geomagnetic storm.

He stopped and waited for satellites to be redirected and my pupils to home in on radio navigation signals, as if a missile to its target, and survive re-entry. How long I wondered was I out of orbit?

Was it seconds, minutes, or had I imagined zoning out?

I returned from wherever my thoughts fled and heard Dr. Sidhu speaking to me. Had I experienced an aura signalling another seizure coming on? What had caused my befuddlement?

*Nine one one, what's your emergency?* Dr. Sidhu's kind eyes appeared to ask.

Hypervigilant senses tuned in, seeking clarity. Then hadn't.

I experienced a temporary shutdown and couldn't articulate any of it to Dr. Sidhu. He waited for my spinning and spiralling mind feverishly dancing the tarantella to slow and be ready to proceed.

Dr. Sidhu, ever mindful, gauged my barometer and modified his content and pacing to prevailing atmospheric conditions.

"I'm not going to beat around the bush, Jocelyn," he said. "There's a lot coming at you. It's a severe condition. It's a big deal. However, there's hope and you're going to get better."

*I was going to get better.* If Dr. Sidhu believed it, maybe I could too. Of all the diagnostic mumbo jumbo that coloured my thinking February 17, 2021, what stuck were Dr. Sidhu's warm hues. His words were life-changing, experience-shifting, and profound. His choice of colours connected with grey matter, and my cognitively impaired black-and-white thinking. I wanted to be certain I wouldn't forget what I'd heard.

"Please Dr. Sidhu, could you repeat that for me? I want to write down what you've just said. I believe that's going to be significant for me to remember."

"Absolutely, Jocelyn."

While he repeated the short matter-of-fact phrases, I

recorded his impactful choice of words in my health diary.

"Dale, do you have any questions about anything you've heard?" Dr. Sidhu asked.

Much to my surprise, he hadn't asked any.

Later, Dale told me he'd been anxious briefly after hearing I would be allowed to drive. He'd witnessed an incredible number of seizures. Dale was more level-headed than I'd been when I was a sleep-deprived, cognitively-challenged soul. But he knew how much I missed the independence that a driver's license provided, and was reassured knowing that he wouldn't be handing the car keys over any time soon.

"I was pleased for you," he said.

I was ecstatic for me!

Ever the optimist, Dale was grateful that we'd been given hope for the first time. That was progress. He wondered where do we go from here? And what steps we'd need to take after the FND diagnosis. But he had confidence we'd be able to handle it. He even headed to one of the websites Dr. Nedd mentioned, he later told me.

"I read a little," Dale offered. But he hadn't scoured the website like a Ph.D. candidate whose thesis, body, and soul depended on grasping each minute detail, as I had. Mastery and comprehension of the website's content mattered to this newly-diagnosed task mistress. Unlike me, Dale focused on the good news. Dale is and always has been my critical infrastructure. He's the bow to my arrow, and compass bearing for my impulsivity.

"You'll be able to drive again. You've had exceptional care. Yes, we've been through a whirlwind, but for the first time we have a plan that's being put in place." Dale's words were a soothing balm.

Dr. Sidhu thanked me again and then complimented me on my determination to strive for wellness.

I asked if I would be seeing him again, hoping that might be the case. He gave me his contact information to pass on to my local psychiatrist in the Comox Valley.

"Goodbye, Jocelyn."

As he exited through the door my soul lurched. Experience made me wary, and I longed to be reassured by continuity of connection and care.

I sat on the bed, still attached by my brain umbilical cord, and overwhelmed didn't even begin to describe what was going on in my mind. I was being discharged first thing tomorrow morning with an unexpected diagnosis that after being described made sense on the surface, but that I didn't truly understand.

*Was FND like what had happened when I'd fallen asleep and the uncertainty of not knowing whether, or not, I'd experience central apnea triggered seizures?*

Would I be okay on the trip home? We'd learned my seizures wouldn't kill me, even though they caused immeasurable distress to everyone in my proximity, and especially me. Was there no rush to help or support me simply because my events weren't neurological, or with physical underpinnings?

What about when I got to Comox? I hadn't been able to walk more than six minutes without having a seizure, or be left alone unattended for months.

I wasn't calm or confident knowing there was so much uncertainty ahead. I'd wanted a diagnosis and clarity but hadn't expected this.

We'd been given hope by specialists. I wanted to lean into Dr. Sidhu's reassurance, but I needed more. I hoped my Saviour, who held and holds my heart, would supply my needs while I had less than sufficient faith.

*Help me God, don't let Satan win. Amen.*

I hadn't been gifted superpowers or a crystal ball. I was fearful, but there was a new spark, and it flickered.

Dale reminded me to plug in and recharge the battery of my Life Alert emergency button. I'd been wearing it when

I arrived at Vancouver General and would need it to be recharged for the trip home. I'd need to remember to call the nurse for help and get that done.

When I asked Dale, after the fact, how he'd felt after each team reported their findings, I needed to sit through an uncomfortable silence with curiosity without interrupting. It was a while until his brows lifted and he turned to face me directly.

"When it sunk in that you were coming home without meds," he said, "I experienced shortness of breath."

I'd had a similar reaction. Had he needed to use his inhalers to prevent an asthma attack? Most likely, yes. I'd never know.

Dale reserved his fears, so as not to add to mine.

What I did learn months later was that Dale had immediately called and talked to our son Keith.

"Keith offered to work remotely from Comox for the first two weeks, and Kristen weeks three and four," Dale told me. It was a practical plan that encouraged calm, his and mine, Keith and Kristen's. It's what Dale does best. It's one of the reasons I said yes when he asked me to be his wife.

Dale stands out and rises above.

~

After supper Dr. Hrazdil dropped in to speak with me. My fingers were racing across my laptop keys composing an email, which when finished would be sent to select few.

Who was it important to tell, and what would I say? Who might be a Nosey Nellie, and how might I diplomatically answer their questions?

"Consider yourself lucky," Dr. Hrazdil said with raised brows. Her expression and tone confirmed I'd been blessed. "Dr. Sidhu made a phone call after seeing you today. He called the neuropsychiatry department at UBC, where he's the head of their psychiatry department."

She'd looked at me quizzically and added, "I don't know what you talked about, but he put a high priority note on your referral and called on your behalf."

That spoke volumes. Dr. Sidhu hadn't just fanned a tiny spark, he'd made sure all three required elements for a successful campfire were taken care of. He ensured my referral had heat (he'd triple checked all the boxes), oxygen (without which my hopes would have been snuffed out), and fuel (he'd called on my behalf).

I could feel the warmth and heat in the dancing flames. Dr. Sidhu made me feel worthy of care and deserving of support. My smile dazzled and twinkled long after camping season ended and campfire's flames were extinguished.

JOCELYN BYSTROM

# CHAPTER TWENTY-THREE

### What Next?

My impish, controlling critic, Bossy Jocie, waited for slivers of vulnerability, then pounced.

*Danger Alert, Danger Alert, Danger Alert*! She'd remind me: *You're not safe*. Skewed code informed my biology after the imp successfully sowed seeds of fear.

I left the SIU with a thimble full of understanding about my new mental health diagnosis. An FND diagnosis only partially provided the insights I'd long been seeking, but certainly provided a strong impetus to reflect on my health, well-being, and diagnostic experience. I wanted still to desperately understand what my body had being trying to tell me all along.

Fueled by Dr. Sidhu's strong belief that I would get better, I dared to believe I'd be able to sew again. I wanted to be confident that there would come a day when I could complete quilting projects I'd begun prior to mixed messages making it impossible to thread the needle on my Bernina sewing machine. After I'd rolled the rotary cutting tool into the index finger of my left hand and bloodied the fabric, I'd stopped playing with fabric. I didn't want to space out and sew over my fingers. Could I now look forward to sewing my way back to a joyful life?

The basic wiring that controlled my nervous system was okay. I thanked God for that. It felt miraculous to have been told that there was nothing neurologically wrong with my brain when I'd believed otherwise for the last seven years.

I was desperate to understand more fully this unexpected diagnosis. Was FND responsible for the engraved terror filed in my amygdala? Would each terrifying seizure recorded in my brain stem arise from the dead zombie-like and continue to cause my muscles to howl, and groan, and jerk, and seize? I hoped the seizures I'd experienced wouldn't haunt me with an apocalyptic return.

I required prerequisite skills to lovingly tend my emotional garden and nurture myself. I wanted to discharge fear and return to a place of safety and calm. A place where my beautiful mind felt tethered, secure, and could trust neural circuitry to send accurate messages.

I wanted to liberate and embrace the full range of emotional expression and be mentored by someone I could trusted to facilitate the healthy and functional aspects of anger, sadness, and fear. Someone who could support me to complete the grieving work I still needed to do. Someone to help smooth the way for me to discharge the inner pain my body still held.

It was my messaging system that was haywire, behaved erratically, and flagged an FND diagnosis. My symptoms were real, not imagined or put on. They paralleled those seen in structural or degenerative diseases like Parkinson's and Alzheimer's, except were caused by functional neurologic disorder.

Historically, FND was perceived as an entirely psychological disorder which caused physical symptoms that were specifically linked to a traumatic incident. Functional symptoms were explained as medical symptoms with no known physical cause. Examples might be weakness or paralysis, tremors or loss of balance, difficulty swallowing or episodes of shaking. These functional symptoms were thought to be explicitly linked to mental illness and caused by stressful life events, both recent and during the developmental years. The medical community don't often look for alternate risk factors and may assume trauma as the primary cause. These may be elements of an FND diagnosis, but they don't provide a full explanation and can also be absent.

Understanding these idiosyncrasies about FND supported wellness for me. Someone may well come up with a scientific theory which will adequately explain why I experienced seizures every day in the weeks up until February 17, and no more February 18, or any day thereafter.

Having both the neurology and psychiatric teams reassure me that my functional symptoms and cognitive decline were indeed exceedingly real and not all in my head was critically important. They were a part of the miracle that helped reduce my anxiety, which in large part seemed to have cause the physiological symptoms I experienced. It was my brain sending and receiving cryptic communications that caused my seizures.

Is it possible, I wondered, that the subconscious mind was aware that I was at a renowned institution, that my brain had been studied by experts in their respective fields, who were in turn certain about their conclusions, and the FND diagnosis that created the extreme shift from a life with seizures to a life journeying to well-being? Could a subconscious awareness and the specialists' confidence in my ability to recover somehow have infused my conscious mind with a different perspective and renewed hope?

~

Was I ignorant and unaware of the basic premise of whole-body wellness at fifty-seven as I left the seizures investigation unit? Yes.

I pondered each day how to explain to others what FND was. I gazed at the laptop I'd purchased in 2007 to begin my master's degree, used daily during my brain health journey through 2021, and saw a useful tool to detail my story.

I was compelled to record a miracle.

~

"You can expect a tapering off of your seizures, Jocelyn."

*Fewer seizures?* That was hard to believe. I'd expected more not less, after ten seizures in quick succession in the past week. I was going home without antiepileptics.

*Why would there be less?*

*What if they were wrong, and more were on the way?* Terrified Jocelyn catastrophized.

Despite all my questions and uncertainty, I was still lighter in my spirit travelling home, lighter than I'd expected to be. The likelihood of psychogenic nonepileptic seizures, or PNES, was high. I was unmedicated and without antiepileptics in my system. When discharged, I was told I could probably expect a gradual improvement of my cognitive abilities. And that, by working with a neuropsychologist the rate of returned cognition might be enhanced.

Whatever it took, I was ready to carry the torch. I hadn't noticed right away, but I was already experiencing greater mental acuity.

There were no seizures en route to the ferry, aboard the vessel, or seated in the car as we crossed the Strait of Georgia and returned to Vancouver Island. We hadn't taken any chances or climbed the stairs to the passenger decks. I was still immunocompromised according to my neuroimmunologist.

There was no rigidity or increased myoclonus after long hours of sitting in the car, as had occurred on most other occasions. We arrived home just after seven in the evening. My body appeared to be content and silenced.

I was grateful to be safely home without incident. We hadn't needed to alert emergency services or explain that I wasn't an epileptic. I was thrilled that there hadn't been a need to call 911.

But bedtime lay ahead, and I hadn't allowed myself to

fall asleep in the car. What would happen when this exhausted girl's head hit the pillow, and my weary body melted into the warmth of familiarity?

I was still wait-listed for a two-day sleep-study, neurologists at the SIU had recommended. The referral was made in hopes of sorting out my dysregulated sleep patterns and experiences of central apnea. I still required support to ensure I could get the seven hours of rest needed to promote optimal health.

What if as I lay horizontal in the cool and darkened room, I became frozen with full-body rigidity, as I had several nights in the SIU, before seizing? Lids drooped and limbs relaxed. Would a brittle tree creak and groan, forecasting a violent storm, and cause shallow roots to be lifted up and out of the ground? Would an unsupported trunk and weighted limbs crash to the forest floor?

I hoped Dale wouldn't sleep peacefully through an incident of silent rigidity. One of the nurses at the SIU hadn't noticed when she'd peeked in. She must have believed that I was fast asleep, leaving the room as silently as she arrived. She hadn't returned till the seizure like a shapeshifter changed from lower case r - rigidity to capital R – and roared with large powerful, repetitive, functional movements. I'd been wide-eyed, rigid, and unable to speak as I watched her leave, and left alone with my fears. Like at five, when I lay awake waiting for Mom to get home from work while the sitter sat somewhere unaware. She'd assumed I was sleeping.

My lack of knowledge about my FND diagnosis sent shivers up and down my spinal cord. I needed a quick fix.

How quickly I'd forgotten in whom I could trust. Rather than ease into sleep after prayer, I sat upright, opened my trusty laptop, and revisited FNDhope.org.

I wanted to be prepared to explain an FND diagnosis to extended family, friends, colleagues, and Nosey Nellie.

I learned at the website that the explanation I provided might vary dependent on who asked. What, if anything, did each need to know, if anything at all?

As I sat in bed avoiding sleep and fearing seizures, I learned that it was my decision. It was my choice of who and what I told anyone about my mental health.

Often, I decided, I would use the "shorter version" I'd found under the FAQ section of the FNDhope.org website. I memorized that one, knowing I'd return to it time and time again.

*"I have a neurological disorder. It's when the brain does not send and receive messages accurately."*

I read and learned that individuals newly diagnosed with FND may find it almost impossible to sum up the physical and emotional pain they've experienced, let alone explain a neurological diagnosis even doctors don't fully understand.

I didn't owe everyone that shuffled by an explanation, not even everyone that asked. "The shortest" definition, I'd kept in my back pocket, ready and waiting for the day I was introduced to nosey Nellie. I'd be ready to explain FND truthfully if Nellie asked:

*I have a neurological disorder.*

~

It was time for rest.

*Lord Jesus, keep me safe through till morning and calm my fear. Amen.*

When I awakened, looked around the room and remembered, it was with a smile.

Still no sign of either rigidity, or nonepileptic seizures. I'd marinated in stress juice before heading to bed and allowed my lids to droop. I awakened able to tally another eight seizure-free hours. We enjoyed a celebratory breakfast and I relaxed, a little.

Through the day I clicked and clicked and clicked to understand the mixed emotions I was experiencing. I read about others with FND, and the stigma they'd faced. Would this also be my experience?

By day's end, I'd surprised myself with a conscious shift, made easier by another fourteen seizure-free hours.

I hadn't considered myself mentally ill, even if I had disorders that affected my mood, thinking, and behavior.

I wouldn't be defined by any traditional definition of mental illness; I was and am so much more than the challenges my brain manages. I'm a capable, strong, loveable individual. I would reframe my story and choose to meet my mental health needs similarly to that of any other body part. It was simply health care I required above the neck.

*The brain was just another body part.* Everyone had a brain and required mental health.

At home, I'd known that I needed additional mental health support to fuel my belief that wellness was possible. Dr. Sidhu wouldn't be there daily to inspire, listen, and reassure a mind that, like a pendulum, swings rhythmically between fear/anxiety and courage/bravery. There were no immediate mental health resources provided right away, or for most of the remainder of 2021. A local psychiatrist pointed me to a website for CCI, the Center for Clinical Innovations based in Western Australia, but it took hard work and initiative to ensure I worked through the assertiveness modules I'd found. Nonetheless, they proved a good place to start while I waited for local supports to be in place. I learned to advocate and ask for the help I deserved and required. Each module helped me to express myself and my point of view in a way that was clearer and more direct, while still respecting the needs of others. I wondered why there weren't medical practitioners who could teach me these supportive skills offered locally, or as part of a progressive mental health curriculum in my community or in our public schools. Couldn't there be a more proactive approach for children who'd missed out on these development social/emotional skills typically learned throughout childhood?

With my Life Alert button fully charged and hanging

around my neck, I continued to count the seizure-free hours rather than sheep.

Each tomorrow was just another day, and an opportunity to choose to continue the necessary hard work to overcome obstacles that now stared me in the face. Unresolved grief after the loss of a treasured career, distress tolerance skills to support myself when I lacked courage in the face of adversity, as well as assertiveness to speak up when needed and found myself overly anxious.

I made a conscious choice to view my recent experiences with FND, and functional symptoms, as a necessary prerequisite for improved skill, strength, and capacity for healthy living. I'd been given a second chance to prioritize and appreciate with gratitude my life, and whatever it took, I wanted to live long and well moving forward.

Each experience provided an invitation and growing awareness of skills I could choose to learn and aim to master to ensure I'd be more assertive, better equipped with improved relational communication, and the impetus to connect more authentically with loved ones. It became increasingly obvious during my brain health journey that my ability to talk about the tough stuff was impaired.

I hadn't intended my emotions to influence or traumatize friends and family, and I wanted to proactively learn skills that would improve my interpersonal communication.

When I felt fear, anger, shame, guilt, envy, jealousy, or sadness in the past, I safely tucked the feelings I couldn't identify, and wasn't certain what to do with away. Buried deep.

It took extreme lengths for my body to reach out and inform me—and in a way I might understand—that I wasn't effectively discharging emotional turmoil.

Functional movement and toxic seizures reminded me that shame, repressed anger, and unresolved grief triggered by a plethora of normally innocuous stimuli were causing me angst. I'd best pay attention with self-compassion and prioritize my health and well-being.

Ironically enough, at fifty-seven, I had too many unwanted letters behind my name.

Jocelyn Bystrom, B.ED, M.Ed., FND, PTSD, OCD, and GAD (generalized anxiety disorder), were now definitively documented in my medical health records, but none of these would define me! I'd asked parents, of my students, through the years, what three adjectives they might use to describe their child to offer me insights as an educator.

I knew now the words that I'd want others to offer if asked to describe me: curious, kind, and humble.

Everybody's experiences with FND are unique, because every unique body responds in its own way. My medical records store data about blood work, lab results, CAT scans, MRIs, and surgeries among others notes medical practitioners have recorded. For example, there'd be record of a C-section (1994), and carpal tunnel surgeries, on both the right and left hands (2007).

Did it really matter that in 2021, they'd added various mental health diagnoses that explained how my body responded to varied experiences, incidents, and misadventures? These additional records ought not to have changed anything much. Other than that, they'd helped create a more vivid picture of my next steps towards whole-body health and well-being.

I chose to conceptualize the stressors in my life differently from here on in. I responded to this new diagnostic information about my needs to effect positive change.

More important than my health records in affecting change were my mindset and relationships. They had the ability to change the trajectory of my day and life whether at home, or at work. I wanted to connect and listen to my body and mind (self-care), as well as invest in others I cared about (other-care). Perhaps if I listened first instead of my default strategy to teach and fix, I'd be more adequately prepared for the life I wanted.

My batteries were incredibly depleted after years of complex physical health investigation and experiences. I took a step back and shifted from being task-focused to prioritizing self-care and my valued relationships instead. I chose to take the time to learn to love myself.

If I got cancer or had MS, I wouldn't blame myself or feel shame about it, so why was it that I was making this qualitative assessment about myself because I have mental health challenges. Society perceives mental health so differently than physical health, and initially with a mental health diagnosis, it's easy to fall victim to societies way of thinking. I've grown and moved away from that kind of thinking, because I'm a good person.

The fact that I have FND, or any of these mental health challenges, does not change the fact that I am a kind human.

~

I was ignorant, unaware, and dazed by my new FND diagnosis those early days yet learned that this is often the case with any new diagnosis. Who wouldn't be in a state of shock after being told your life was about to be forever changed by a physical, mental, relational, or spiritual-health determination? The unexpected baffled me, as it would have anyone.

I was grateful for my diagnosis. I longed for restored health more than just about anything. I deserved to be well and was worthy of the support I needed. If anything was going to stand in my way, it wouldn't be my own ignorance or attitude.

Negativity had no place and would create consequences which would get in the way of the personal empowerment I wanted. Secrets had no place in my life. I wanted to be authentic and to learn how to communicate assertively as I examined the advantages and disadvantages of disclosing that I had a mental illness. I couldn't do it all on my own.

Initially I was in a state which could be best described as disbelief. I had a mental illness. Really! How could I have a severe psychiatric illness, and how had it caused such extreme physical symptoms. It was mind-boggling.

I was overwhelmed by the limited and varied information available. I'd wanted to talk to someone rather than read online. My experience of an FND diagnosis was mine alone and will have been different from anyone else's. When first told of my FND diagnosis perhaps the most significant piece, was that I embraced the diagnosis. It wasn't life shortening or terminal. And thanks to Dr. Sidhu, I believed I could get well if I chose to act and complete the hard work required to journey to wellness.

You don't recover from mental illness; my goal wasn't to be cured. I wanted wellness, and it was within my grasp.

Wholeness was what I required. I looked ahead with optimism and believed I would be given resolute strength to make use of the gifts God had already provided. I had so much to look forward to... the rest of my joyful life.

More good news soothed my soul. I'd picked up a novel I began reading over a year earlier and put down indefinitely when my eyes couldn't track between the lines of text. I was now able to read for pleasure without impairment. Hallelujah! That was a definite game changer.

I imagined my way through the cycle I knew my mind required to prepare for what was to come, rather than being ever alert for risk. I needed to do something to move stress and fear through my body, complete the cycle and return to a state of resilience and discharge any residual inner pain.

I began to reflect on my most recent stressors, debilitating seizures that terrified me, and what that felt like in my body. I wanted to eliminate any threats to my physiological being. How could I focus on what completed the cycle and return to a homeostasis? What evidence and data could I look back on to challenge illness, and be well?

My most important factors seemed to be sleep, creativity, nutrition, and exercise, as well as to nurture my spiritual health. I made sure I was in bed by ten o'clock and that my reading light was off shortly thereafter.

I drew walking routes on a neighborhood map, left notes about which one I was headed out on, and when I'd expected to return. Dale wasn't keen on me heading out alone, but it wasn't his decision. It was mine. I was taking back my life.

I wore the Life Alert button, which was Dale's nonnegotiable condition, and started with a fifteen-minute daily walk to see how it would go. I'd listened to important pearls of wisdom offered by medical practitioners that I trusted and was mindful to start small.

Family and friends had learned and known that I set the bar high for myself, and consistently strove to reach great heights.

Don't increase your pace or the intensity of any workout more than once every two weeks, mindful me voiced, she'd listened and reminded impulsive me. I'd let my body take its time as it learned to respond and build capacity before increasing my exercise goals.

*Otherwise, you'll end up with seizures!* I reminded Jocelyn version 57.1.

In typical Jocelyn fashion, I wanted to be as fit again and feel as strong as I was briefly in 2019. At the time, I'd known my physical body was in decline, but not why. I'd decided to spend the year becoming as fit as possible so that if the decline continued it would be from a peak level of fitness. I'm not the patient type. Was I ready to listen to my body, rather than Bossy Jocie?

Dale and I celebrated seven days seizure-free. There ought to have been a parade with a celebrated parade marshal.

Ms. FND 2021 was in the house. Dale couldn't believe it, nor could I. With 168 symptom-free hours, our joy factor septupled.

"Dale," I said, "I've been gifted a miracle."

He concurred those seven days seizure-free seemed miraculous, though he wasn't as easily convinced as I. He continued to seek scientific explanations that explained the why in a way his analytical brain could understand.

Intelligent brains needed to know. Why had I experienced seizures every day and right up until the last day at the seizure unit, and none since? There was no tapering of symptoms, just a sudden miraculous stop.

He was appreciative, but not ready to return my Life Alert button, just yet.

He knew that I faith, and believed, but it wasn't as obvious to him yet. It had only been a week.

I felt differently. My cognition was 100 percent restored. I hadn't experienced a single myoclonic jerk. There were no functional symptoms whatsoever. I hadn't experienced a regulated body in seven years. Now, all was well, it seemed. It was like hearing the clarity of a definitive diagnosis had cured me and cleared away the stress of non-understanding, although I knew better. There is no cure for FND.

I began remembering details, no longer needed to ask others to repeat themselves after my brain hadn't coded information, and there was further evidence of functional symptoms.

I believed it. I'd experienced a miracle.

There didn't seem to be a scientific explanation that could explain the sudden, instantaneous changes between February 17 and February 18, 2021. Although I still wondered about a scientific rationale because Dale seemed so certain there must be one.

By the end of March, I was certain beyond a doubt. I felt alive! I felt confident, and I planted the seed about being ready to drive.

"I'm not ready to hand you the keys," Dale said. I hadn't even asked; he simply needed to assert himself. I respected Dale, and his not being ready just yet.

My counsellor reiterated Dale's wait and see opinion. I needed to be patient not only with myself, but with Dale.

"He's experienced considerable trauma too," she reiterated.

*Each time I'd seized had he worried that I'd stop breathing and not start again?* I would cut Dale some slack, and anyone else who may have been traumatized as they'd witnessed my seizures. I needed to mindfully reconsider events I'd experienced through the lens of others around me, which I hadn't been able to do while I was moving through them in an elevated state of hyperarousal.

I listened and attempted to tolerate delays in what I was able to do, but patience has never been my middle name. I desperately wanted to be back to work, able to go out and about, and to drive. So badly, I wanted to drive!

I called and made an in-person doctor's appointment for June 24, 2021, to ask questions about next steps, and to receive another's perspective on how realistic my goals were.

I knew in my heart I could drive safely. I hadn't risked it though because I'm legalistic. I'd wait till my doctor agreed and gave me the green light. I wouldn't jeopardize anyone's health or safety. But that was no longer the point. I believed I was ready.

At the three-month mark, even Dale couldn't explain the facts away. Something miraculous had happened. After four thousand three hundred and sixty-eight hours I continued to be seizure and symptom free.

It takes time to understand and accept a mental health diagnosis.

What kind of a miracle can shift perception, and had enabled me to trust a higher power and believe? What was the turning point or paradigm shift that prepared me to understand that I didn't need to be in control, and in fact hadn't been all along? In relinquishing control to my Heavenly Father, He mercifully lifted the burden of stress and trauma from my body.

*Isn't that how faith works?* I questioned.

Perhaps there's an interplay between faith, trust, and healing. Had I subconsciously realized what was required and believed all things were possible with God? Was surrender the prerequisite for wholeness and well-being?

As I considered my life through the lens of a lovingly handcrafted fabric, I wondered, what had happened at the intersections of woven threads? Was not one but more than one integral thread pulled and loosened? Perhaps that's why the fabric of my life quite literally fell apart.

Could the answers lay between the warp and weft of yarns interlaced at right angles when one or more are yanked out unexpectedly?

With conscious acceptance of faith, can there be a scientific override of brain dysfunction? Humanly speaking, I'd thought it impossible. But I'd learned, in Sunday School, that "With God everything is possible." (Matthew 19:26)

*Be gentle on yourself, Jocelyn. Take the time you need to heal and process the traumatic stress of what you've just experienced.*

I may appear well, but there'd been a significant number of traumatic seizures layered on top of unexpected life events. There would be hard work and struggles ahead. Functional neurologic disorder isn't a disease; it can't be cured. It would be with me for life.

My miracle wasn't a miraculous healing. My miracle was the miraculous gift of a life worth living, knowing I'm held and have hope.

The best news?

*It's treatable.* I could get better and look forward with hopeful expectation.

JOCELYN BYSTROM

# PART FIVE

## SEASON OF GROWTH

# CHAPTER TWENTY-FOUR

### Care Above and Below the Neck

Most people are too busy to notice the gentle caress of the wind on their skin, or the warmth of the sun at their back. I know I was for far too long. I was too busy doing rather than being, and perpetually focused on the completion of my to-do list. Efficient, intelligent thinking was hijacked by my instinctual brain any time my body perceived threat or danger. Now, I wanted to slow and delight in the presence of light filtering through the leaves and canopy overhead.

Everyone with a new diagnosis of any kind deserves respectful, collaborative care and follow-up treatment options explained, so as not to become more overwhelmed. When I hadn't understood aspects of my FND diagnosis, I realized it was my responsibility to seek the clarifications I required. There's a definite need to assert yourself as you navigate a new health diagnosis.

Follow-up care and treatment options, like the seven-year diagnostic journey, were inadequate. If my experience of an FND diagnosis was typical, then our health care system is indeed broken. No medical professional would diagnose a life-altering cancer, Parkinson's, or multiple sclerosis diagnosis with nothing more than a referral to head to the World Wide Web.

It took nine months to hear back about an opening in a community health based dialectical behavioural therapy (DBT) group. It took twelve months until Dr. Sidhu's prioritized referral was successful, and I was able to meet with a neuropsychiatrist.

I required and deserved more.

I needed a mental health mentor who I could call for reassurance and security when functional behaviours were activated in the part of the brain scientists know as the limbic system. I'd trusted that support was on its way for my cross-wired amygdala. If I hadn't experienced a miracle and needed to cope with continued daily seizures and functional symptoms, my story may have ended very differently.

My prefrontal cortex—essential to my ability to accomplish goals and self-determination—was being directed by motor and cognitive functions that received cryptic code. Learning this after going home made me wonder if my vast neural network looped back and influenced my central and peripheral nervous system, causing seizures.

Was the scientific explanation for what had seemed a miraculous shift a result of Dr. Sidhu's reassurances that calm and serenity were possible? Had *this* been enough to reverse the two-way neural loop that wasn't functioning properly?

There may have been a significantly different diagnostic journey had my GP known that FND, and functional symptoms, are similarly the result of a dynamic two-way communication between brain structures and the body. Dynamic yet dysfunctional, it seemed.

Could an FND diagnosis similarly be the result of a dynamic two-way communication between brain structures and the body, like the way childhood behaviours influenced functional behaviours in the classroom?

Could it be that our health-care infrastructure, with its highly specialized medical model for brain and body, is getting in the way of whole-body wellness and big-picture thinking? Research on polyvagal theory suggested that dynamic two-way communication between the brain and the body influences our mental state and prejudices our perception of the environment. What did this mean for me with FND?

My autonomic nervous system and emotional regulation shaped the way I moved through the world and interacted with others. It all began in my biology. I needed to be able to flexibly move between various states in the autonomic hierarchy. I needed to leave a state of thinking that the world was a scary unwelcoming place and get to a state where I believed that the world was filled with possibility—where I'd be assured, I was connected, capable and loved.

I learned throughout 2021 that my ability to self-regulate comes from being safely held in relationship with another, and that, for me, well-being is found in the connections between myself, my body, my spirit, and others in my world. When I can co-regulate with others, it's more likely that I'll experience safety and connection and find a healthy landscape where growth and restoration from functional symptoms is possible.

*Aha!* When I couldn't return to a state of grounded, mindful curiosity, I'd been stuck in a dissociative, shutdown manner, and I seized. I needed a sense of safety, and my lack of capacity to respond was impaired by my inability to communicate and assert my needs.

It took learning body-awareness techniques that were part of cognitive behavioral therapy (CBT) and practicing dialectical behavioural therapy (DBT) skills to help me move out of a state where my body constantly expressed itself with functional behaviours. I needed to return to a more embodied state, deepen my awareness of my breath, and activate my sympathetic nervous system. Only then was I eventually able to return to a more playful level of arousal and restorative surrender, which created calm to my supercharged nervous system.

I needed a GP who could answer yes when asked, "Are you FND aware?"

Had he been aware, he might have recognized my symptoms and functional behaviours as characteristic of FND and known to prescribe CBT and DBT rather than antiepileptics.

I hadn't had the skill, capacity, or mental energy to do the advocacy work I needed to do for myself between 2013–2020. I'd needed answers and support that would have helped me assertively communicate and describe my internal life. Instead, I was referred from one specialist to the next, none of whom had observed the mind-body connection of my functional symptoms or specialized in mental health.

After my FND diagnosis, I was filled with compassion for others who continue to struggle with their mental health. The inadequacies of extended health care plans offered by employers don't adequately cover counselling and therapists for those in need.

It may be different elsewhere, but I constantly ran into the challenge of finding the specific type of support and collaborative practitioners that I required.

I found it tough to navigate a health care system, where the status quo abandons individuals with mental health challenges. I was left alone, and in double jeopardy. I was vulnerable and left to manage my own health and well-being while cognitively compromised by post-traumatic stress that caused anxiety, compulsive behavior, and functional symptoms. Long waiting lists for publicly funded mental health programming exponentially taxed my already maxed-out mind and body.

None of us are born with the ability to control our behaviours. Instead, we acquire skills to manage our behaviour over time through empathetic sentient relationships. I was a kid who didn't receive the parental nurturing I needed.

I hadn't had a father eager to participate in tough conversations, give me positive feedback, or even show up. I missed out on parenting that provided resources for ongoing verbal, and social-emotional development. Mom provided both physical and spiritual nurturance, but I had soul-ache. I longed for someone to help me develop the practices of self-care, self-protection, and self-love. The damage was done before meeting Dale, as his love and care were never in question.

I missed out on that special someone, who delighted in meeting me consistently with caring, regard, and interest. Mom loved me in the best ways she knew how, but I missed out on the parental resources to teach me safe ways to release anger, or to honour tears as a way of releasing hurt. I lacked a safe refuge.

My functional symptoms disappeared February 18, 2021, but invisible mental health symptoms had not. I may have appeared fine, though I still required support to thrive with FND.

One of the most important ways I was able to acquire care was to invite willing practitioners, who may or may not be FND aware, to come alongside me with curiosity and compassion.

Functional behaviours, I learned, can diminish when our physiological and emotional needs are addressed. Another possible scientific explanation.

*Aha!*

That was exactly what Dr. Sidhu did for me. His strength and assurances provided me the prerequisite building blocks for a regulated physiological state. Perhaps my miracle was being gifted personalized care by knowledgeable specialists able to help build a foundation of calm. Drs. Hrazdil and Nedd had restored my physiological state with "big-picture" thinking and clarity when they reminded me, "There's nothing neurologically wrong with your brain." Dr. Sidhu capped that with his certainty. *I was going to get better.*

He acknowledged that my symptoms were very real, and characteristic of a *"severe condition." He believed me!*

Simultaneously he reassured my soul's ache, when he'd said, *"There's hope."* That day, February 17, a day when my needs were finally addressed, I was tethered. Heavenly stars were aligned for my miracle, and God answered my cry.

I built my house on rock-solid ground but hadn't learned the skills essential to build an unshakeable, social-emotional foundation. When the winds howled, and the earth quaked, my house couldn't stand secured. At times my foundation seemed solid, but alternately was shaken, or somewhere in between. Traumatic incidents left me unnerved, bewildered, and seizing.

I longed to thrive rather than survive my residual inner turmoil. I wanted to be active again and out and about in the world, believing I was capable, connected, and able to achieve my goals and dreams.

Mid-pandemic I sought to reactivate my weary body. I was shocked to be turned away from participating in an outdoor fitness class. A fitness challenge that was advertised as: *An opportunity to get fit with friends and training partners for moral support.* I was excited and signed up impulsively, knowing that if there were others to keep me going and active it would be more fun. The class advertised: *No matter what your starting point, we have fitness plans to suit your needs.*

Apparently not, if you have multiple mental health diagnoses. I believe that's called stigma.

The class was well within my physical capabilities, and I'd truthfully documented my newly diagnosed mental health conditions (plural). I was turned away with an apology. They were sorry but felt they couldn't risk having someone with multiple health diagnoses, who might not be covered by their insurance if something happened to me during the training.

I voluntarily told them on my registration about my health diagnoses and wasn't ashamed to record diagnostic information I'd waited seven years to receive. Had I kept these mental health diagnoses secret I'm certain they would have welcomed my registration and participation.

Getting fit is seemingly only a treatment option if you have a single physiological diagnosis, like cancer or diabetes. If I'd simply told them I had FND, which they wouldn't likely know much about, or had not explained that it was a mental health diagnosis, would I have been good to go? What exactly made them feel afraid? Were they worried my anxiety or obsessive-compulsive behaviour might get in the way of my ability to run?

I refused to let this attitude or fear get in my way. It didn't seem fair or kind. And so, I exercised alone.

I had a fierce determination to be well, strong, and fit. I was able to do it solo.

Of course, it would have been much more fun to get fit with like-minded peers who shared similar fitness goals. Instead, Ollie, my faithful fitness fur-buddy cheered me along my path to fitness.

How many individuals have returned home after learning of an FND diagnosis without required and timely follow-up mental health support? I bet it's not a small number.

On June 3, I seized the opportunity and risked everything. I publicly shared what I didn't want to become a secret. I wasn't ashamed and hadn't done anything to cause or deserve FND. And so, I posted to social media: "My name is Jocelyn Bystrom, and I struggle with my mental health." I became an advocate for what I wished I'd been able to find before I started having migraines, myoclonic jerks, and seizures. I posted and blogged about FND and what I'd learned, so that others might read with curiosity, and know what I hadn't.

All of it, all the information I posted initially about FND was acquired from the two websites specialists at the SIU had recommended I check out the day they'd sent me home.

For me, healing took time and required that I courageously ask for help. To ask, and not receive imperative support was jarring. I was supported by family and an increasingly large community of friends, colleagues, and individuals online, but I began seeing common denominators in comment threads about mental health, and particularly about FND.

My created website, writeradvocatejocelynb.com, started getting subscribers almost immediately. I joined several online FND communities and wasn't shocked to read a wide array of comments written by a diverse group of individuals worldwide, who continued to struggle with unexplained symptoms while waiting for support. I started small and hoped to gain a following on social media. Perhaps they could read short posts of one to three minutes max reading time . . . and I could help others who struggled like I had without an FND aware community of medical professionals. My platform increased exponentially after I was approached and invited to share my story by podcast host Monica Parkin, on her program, *Juggling Without Balls*.

Parkin speaks to individuals who juggle relationships, kids, aging parents, work, dating, school, health, and more. She invited me to speak on the topic of mental health. I was surprised to learn that our episode, titled "Mental Health Matters with Jocelyn Bystrom," had a record high number of listeners. Comments I received as I started telling my story were heartwarming and inspired me to continue my mental health advocacy goals. As I shared my struggles with mental health, I was pleasantly surprised that it was also therapeutic and healing. I wasn't alone. There were others out there like me, and lots of them. I may have "very rare normal" epileptiform-appearing spike and wave discharges on my EEGs according to specialists, but like everyone else, I needed mental health care to meet my body's needs.

*Are we a society that accepts the status quo for the provision of mental health care and support when change is necessary?*

Recording my story also unexpectedly improved my well-being. Writing helped discharge memories of the terror I'd experienced along my tumultuous diagnostic journey. Writing about my seizures was incredibly difficult, but the weight of each seizure lifted each time I put pen to paper.

As I wrote, reread, and revised my story I was able to capture my experiences and begin to process each. I was able to consider each event and incident through a new lens, without fear. I began to process experiences I hadn't been able to discharge or grieve. I was finally ready to talk about the tough stuff.

It wasn't any single incident that had happened to me. I hadn't witnessed murder or sheltered fearfully in a war zone. It was what happened inside me following each traumatic incident that left indelible inscriptions on neural pathways. Each time I'd needed to leave a significant relationship behind, wasn't able to express my emotions, needed to move from one community to the next, or find a new best friend was recorded.

It was what happened inside of me that caused soul-ache: my dad abandoning his parenting responsibility, not hearing words of affirmation, or receiving emotional nurturing. It was unresolved grief after yearly layoffs, and then the big whammy, the loss of my treasured teaching position and having not a single person speak in defense of me when my professional integrity was questioned. Somewhere through it all, I lost my ability to trust that others had my back, and that I was held.

In a state of complete desperation, engraved terror filed in my amygdala, developing new neural pathways. My amazing and intelligent brain knew that by sending out mixed up messages I'd seize, and then practiced and practiced and practiced until it mastered the art of complex daily seizures. I seized, and then seized again and again, and again. Perhaps my neural networks and pathways wanted to please and perfect their survival instincts. Would anyone be surprised to learn that my brain retrained itself to achieve excellence when it came to my survival instincts?

My intelligent brain perfected a way of sending mixed-up, erroneously coded neural messages and mastered seizures, like an Olympic gold medalist. Could my mind have created erroneous code and remembered to run that sequence through neural networks causing central apnea and seizures? Foolish me—I can think of far easier and less distressing ways to be seen, heard, and voice my body's need for care and required supports.

I didn't want anyone to experience the immensity of despair that seized me each time a medical practitioner implied, "It's all in your head." A thoughtless remark that wounded my soul and further distressed the girl in the mirror already struggling with her unmet needs.

So easily the message could have been articulated compassionately by saying:

*Your physical symptoms are indeed real Jocelyn. They may be the result of a condition known as FND, or functional neurologic disorder. Symptoms can occur when the brain sends mixed-up messages to the body, but there's hope. Treatment is available, and I believe you can get better.*

It was true: It all started in my head. My brain is protected and sheltered there. My head also houses a complex organ that controls my thoughts, memories, emotions, breathing, temperature, hunger, and every other process that regulates my body. It regulated my senses and motor skills as I seized too.

Our brains are also an enclosed storage space where inner pain is held captive after being hijacked by survival instincts. When I was treated by medical practitioners who appeared disinterested, lacked empathy, or stigmatized the importance of mental health care, they sabotaged my health and wellness.

I was told my discharge paperwork from the SIU would be forwarded to practitioners and specialists. Had those who received my medical records taken the time to read and learn about a little-known mental health diagnosis that over time exacted huge costs?

Or, as I imagined, was my paperwork filed by an efficient administrative assistant? Would my records remain filed until an overworked, exhausted family doctor or medical practitioner saw my name come up in whichever calendar app they used for the appointment I booked online? Would we even have time to review my health records during my ten-minute routine appointment? Certainly, ten minutes wasn't enough time to think "big picture."

My appointments with my GP, soon after the FND diagnosis, were typically telehealth appointments, necessitated by the start of the global pandemic in 2020. It's difficult to read facial cues and body language, or to see physical restoration and realize cognitive reclamation on video. Might they presume I'd recovered enough?

Would my doc ask pertinent questions relating to my health and well-being, and take the time for a mental health check-in?

I trusted God, and knew He'd gifted me with intelligence. I couldn't solely rely on an overburdened, broken public health care system that required change. It was time. I decided to speak up, to plant seeds for change, and to become a more active and collaborative participant in my health care. I'd need to speak up about my mental health and anything I happened to be struggling with. My GP's good, but she can't read minds.

There is a dire need for widespread, mental health education, and access to mental health support in every community.

How could I best support local mental health agencies already prioritizing and advocating mental health and wellness. As an educational leader and mental health advocate my hope was to prioritize changes within my control when possible.

As of 2023, over 8 billion people populate planet Earth, and each one of us requires health care above the neck, for a precious and complex organ sheltered there.

I was grateful for the many who provided me extraordinary care, but simultaneously angered by the inconsistencies of access to mental health care, support, and education for everyone.

I wanted to be part of something bigger than myself and participate in advocacy efforts for individuals experiencing undiagnosed functional symptoms as well as associated mental health challenges. How might I create transparent conversations about FND, a relatively unknown and likely highly underdiagnosed mental health condition worldwide.

*If I chose courage over fear, others might also.* Future medical students and practitioners could crack the code (stigma) and watch for functional symptoms, which may have an underlying mental health underpinning. Medical practitioners could be taught the cipher and to watch for instances where the brain may have stored the body's trauma.

Together we can support individuals struggling with FND and unlock secrets recorded in invisible ink. We're stronger together.

~

Encrypted messages continued to swirl and spiral in the deep crevices of my mind's eye throughout 2021. I wanted to give each emotion a voice. I wanted to talk about FND and plant seeds for change, acceptance, and growth.

My GP was surprised to learn of my FND diagnosis.

I was excited to be headed back to work although cautiously optimistic I wouldn't be on the receiving end of any work-place stigma following my diagnosis. I hoped that there would be others like me, who supported mental health initiatives and education, and like me, at times struggle with complex health.

Mental health care isn't optional. The incremental costs of neglect are exponentially larger than that of prevention. We can educate ourselves about mental health first aid and cheer on stigma fighters who advocate for mental health supports. I'm hopeful that more individuals will choose to listen with curiosity and without judgement to colleagues, friends, and family members who are perhaps doing everything in their power to take hold of their mind and create calm.

Vulnerable children, adolescents, young adults, new parents, employees, teachers, doctors, leaders, colleagues, inmates, politicians, the unhoused or sleeping rough, are *all* in need of mental health care and may continue to struggle without adequate support.

WE ALL NEED mental health care!

How long must we shelter alone without a foundation of safety and calm?

I didn't need to be alone with grief, loss, pain, and fear.

I believe I am not the only one out there with unexplained physical symptoms that scientists and doctors can't explain.

I'm wired for understanding. I may be a butterfly with a broken wing, and faulty habits of thinking, but I've shed the blinders and acknowledged the hard facts. I required mental health supports to learn to express and assert myself proactively. I lacked the social-emotional intelligence to respond with curiosity and a nonjudgmental attitude. I struggled and continue to struggle with my mental health.

I'm not alone. Eight billion people strong can advocate for health care we all require, above and below the neck.

I ended up imprisoned by fear and shame, needlessly when an awareness of mental health first aid could have prevented functional symptoms. I have theories about others who may be suffering with functional symptoms, and undiagnosed FND. I suspect others, who seek attention in all the wrong places and in inappropriate ways, without required supports they deserved, land themselves in our prison systems. I speculate that children, who don't receive adequate care, lack the foundational elements of emotional regulation, and without firm attachments, lose hope. It's easy to lose hope. I did.

My experiences are my own, as are my opinions. They may differ significantly from others with FND, or not.

I wasn't traumatized by receiving a mental health diagnosis. Quite the opposite was true. Whatever experiences or triggers have caused an individual's neural and limbic systems to be dysregulated, every individual struggling with FND deserves to be heard, treated with respect, and believed.

I needed words of affection to thrive. Every individual's needs are unique, and all deserve respectful, collaborative health care.

I learned to trust and was changed for the better by FND. Fear taught me how to take care of and love myself enough to advocate for the care and support I deserved all along.

Like when Saul encountered Jesus on the road to Damascus, I cried out: *Lord, who'll believe in me?*

Familiar surroundings can be transformed. I experienced a quiet perceptual shift and illumination after my FND diagnosis.

Fog lifted and patches of sun shone through the canopy as I walked, then jogged, and at last was able to run beneath the open sky where sun streamed down between fluttering leaves and nourished me. The gentle breeze refreshed me, and I learned to delight in the sanctuary of the North-East Woods.

I needed to believe I would be held. That I'd be carried while the weight of stigma alarmed and frightened me. I needed to trust that until I was strong enough to become my own best friend and love myself, that girl in the mirror, He'd carry me. I wanted wholeness and wellness.

I hadn't known how to tend my emotional garden and was a people-pleaser constantly hoping to measure up. I was enough and worthy; I just didn't trust. That's changed.

Vivid memories provide ample evidence that I was loved all along. I hadn't loved that girl I saw staring back at me in the mirror. She was waiting to hear that she was enough, worthy, and loved.

Now, I wanted to give her that, and more.

"I'm fine." It's what I'd said but hadn't meant. There must be others like me who at three, thirteen, twenty-three, and fifty-three haven't trusted themselves to express and acknowledge their full spectrum of emotions. I hadn't met many who waited or listened for a fuller answer, as they'd carried on their way. I vowed after I was diagnosed to look deeper into each pair of eyes and question the truth and validity when I heard, "I'm fine."

I hadn't known that I required all my emotions. I believed it was shameful to express anger, sadness, guilt, and fear. I hadn't checked the facts when I needed to or discharged distorted thoughts or judgemental beliefs.

Instead, I buried unwanted emotion. Not a strategy I'd recommend. It didn't work out well for me. I taught students about healthy and functional aspects of emotion while mine lay fallow and uncultivated. I had blinders as I taught social-emotional skills I didn't have myself. Had anyone noticed the discrepancy between what I practiced and preached, and simply chosen not to hold me accountable? I forgave that girl.

Light shines hope into all our dark corners.

I'd needed to know then that anger, sadness, and fear are complex responses linked to a person's internal state and involuntary physiological responses to objects, situations, and individuals. I'd collected all the prerequisite sensory information, but missed out on that shrewd sixth sense that could decipher encrypted code and unlock me when I found myself stuck.

Now, I am finally ready to participate in the quieter rhythms of life. To capture the essence and warmth of the sun rise, embrace a summer rain shower, and delight in heaven-sent signs of spring. The darkened haze that had filled my mind and kept me stuck in the emptiness of winter seeing nothing beyond black, white, and shades of grey, finally lifted.

The ephemerality of intense light that blessed me February 17, signalled renewal. It enabled me to slow and take the needed time to notice, listen, and breathe.

I wasn't home alone as I'd thought. Belief, like an awareness of colour filling a canvas, required a perceptual shift. I could choose to adjust the lens and witness others through a more diverse palette of hues, tones, and textures. I chose to trust more fully each day that I was loved. That I am held.

As I found the courage to trust, the hard work of asserting myself seemed more manageable, and the relational intimacy I sought prompted me to choose courage over fear. I was poised and ready for growth.

*Jesus, tune my eyes and ears to your presence in my daily life so that my heart and vision are transformed. Give me the patience and perseverance required to rejoice as this season of darkness ends, and You light the way forward. Because I will fear again, and that's okay.*

Fear, has its purpose. I see that now.

*Spirit of Light, morning presence, meet me as I greet each new day. You were there in the city of rose-coloured reflective glass, and painted love and light during pandemic living with mirrored love and light across the City of Vancouver.*

*You found me near and far from home. In you I found rest and calm as I sensed your love reflected in the glass. I had a little faith. You planted a desire for more.*

Illumination and radiance shone through a moody fog and vibrant colours invited me to anchor in His metallic-hued embrace.

God reawakened my strength to draw what lay buried deep up from the bottom of a dark well. He brought light to emergent needs seeking release.

I dialled 911, in prayer.

He'd held me in my struggles while I was lost in a labyrinth of fear and uncertainty, seasoned me with curiosity and emboldened me to speak up, and out, when I felt afraid.

Weary lids were opened and equipped for each precious day of life.

# CHAPTER TWENTY-FIVE

### A Tree Needs

June 2021—I emerge into the light a seedling under the canopy of endless blue peeking through a kaleidoscope of green. Warmth embraces me and I am held. Light streams from heaven to touch the earth, providing nurture to tender fresh shoots of innocence. A thin-barked, young dogwood reaches with longing to be conjoined to another. Her limbs outstretched, braid together, seeking, while her roots thirst for nutrients at the edge of the forest, sheltered by the majestic Douglas firs native to the landscape.

A careless man left embers unattended that charred a young sapling's fragile identity and fledgling roots and scarred her tiny flower cluster and petal-like smile. Still maturing, she experienced losses that rearrange her world. The sensitive Pacific dogwood is easily stressed because of its shallow root system.

Like any other plant, I required air, sun, water, soil, nutrients, and care.

A tree needs carbon dioxide from air while I needed oxygen and loving affirmation. Seeking love and nourishment, she inhaled in need of deep cleansing breaths. I rarely thought about air until it hadn't flowed easily. Panic then penetrated my every fibre.

Similarly, God penetrated thickened bark and embraced me even when I was unaware. His compassion cost nothing. It nourished and satisfied a hunger within me as I breathed in slowly. Inhaling through nostrils that longed to meet emotional developmental milestones and to no longer practice emotional withholding.

I wanted to trust and love unconditionally.

I counted the inhale. *One, two, three, four*, then held the breath... *one, two*... before exhaling for seven: *one, two, three, four, five, six, seven.*

It was tough to slow my breath on the exhale. I repeated inhaling gently and deeply, then exhaled slowly and purposefully. Was this a more natural rhythm like trust?

When I was mindful, nourishing breath, like trust was possible. When central apnea impeded, I was frozen with fear and trust vanished. Anxiety ruled my heart when I was terrified. Love was the air I breathed in when I couldn't reach out on the exhales. Dale was the air I'd needed as I seized. Filling and fuelling. Dale was ever-present and always has my back.

Like a tree that creates oxygen as a by-product of a chemical reaction, love's maturity authored a new freedom to choose courage, assert myself, and bloom.

Living water and fertile ground where I could become deeply rooted, were provided by the majesty of the Creator.

I can breathe deeply. I've been gifted a miracle.

A tree needs energy from sunlight, as she does for human health and well-being. I benefit from the sun's ability to generate the production of vitamin D, support bone health, lower blood pressure, prevent disease, and promote good mental health. Without sunlight and airflow through the canopy, the youthful sapling struggles to attain essential elements for healthy growth and development, and her leaves become dry and brittle. Light green on a continuum towards brown and expedited leaf loss. She's susceptible to invasion. Pests and diseases infiltrate her taxed roots, trunk, and soul. Without proper nurture and care, over time, she withers.

A tree needs water to transport nutrients and sugars from the soil, while she needs living water to flush out waste, regulate body temperature and help the brain function efficiently. She needs living water and safe shelter from life's storms. A place where she's rooted, protected, and safe. A home where she can confidently trust for provision, and be skilled with confidence and assertiveness, and mentored to thrive under the canopy of heaven and the dark, speckled starlit sky. She's Home, in the shade of the majestic Douglas fir at the edge of the woods.

~

Research tells me a newly transplanted dogwood requires somewhere between four to ten gallons of water each week during its first growing season. Trees need air and water; I need hydration and life-giving breath. When it hasn't rained for several weeks, I'll need to check on her and see if she needs a drink.

In 2021, she experienced severe thirst during a hot, dry summer on Vancouver Island. She needed nitrogen, phosphorus, and potassium carried through to her roots and carbon dioxide during a season of raging forest fires, intense heat, and little rain. She required extra TLC from her counsellor, a therapist, her care-partners, and friends while she took responsibility to ensure she exercised and fed herself a healthy diet suited to her needs and well-being.

A tree needs soil, while she needs fertile ground to thrive. I picked a location for my dogwood where I'd be able to admire her through our living room window. I researched to find specifics on how to transplant her successfully. My chosen tree would live its life in this hole, and I needed to find out what depth to plant her. This hole would also be the ultimate resting place for an artifact symbolic of losses I've endured and mourn. I would bury the letter that had caused her soul harm here.

A tree needs nutrients and care, while she needs supportive care, without stigma. Trees need a gentle pruning. As do I. Leaves on a dogwood curl, an essential protective reaction to stress the tree feels, which are a result of storms, danger, and uncertainty.

When a child's emotional needs for wellness went unmet, tender roots were pulled and transplanted, repeatedly. New buds were damaged by unexpected frost, the weight of storms, and a mother's silence.

A little pruning cleared away deadwood that was holding her back. She learned to let go of distorted and negative thoughts. Instead of turning away, pushing down or avoiding grief, which deprived her of wholesomeness, she learned to acknowledge that a significant part of herself had now changed, and that considering this, there could be love after loss.

Major pruning, with supportive intervention from counsellors, and a psychiatrist, ensured she had time to process her lived experiences, and communicate then swim through grief's waves.

She learned to hold space and be present for what was going on in her own heart with kindness and care. She wanted to bear with and come alongside others who might experience similar grief and choose to be uncomfortable alongside and hold space while they were being pounded by enormous waves. It's what she'd needed and appreciated. With gratitude, her family, friends, and worship community did just that. They listened, held space, and helped her make room for her heart.

I know now I deserve care, healing, and restoration I needed previously to thrive. With support and applications of slow-release fertilizer regularly to release nutrients into the soil, experienced trauma therapists prepared to listen. With supportive care-partners and a strong personal motivation for wellness, I am positioned to not only thrive, but bloom. Aware of the need to advocate and acquire the care I deserve; I'm learning to assert myself with kindness.

A childlike species, I was transient, rafting, and longing to be naturalized. Thirty rings circled my seed, when with Dale, I became rooted and secure in the Comox Valley. Here my heart and dogwood can be at home. With abundant space, and a nurturing community, I am poised to thrive with fresh air, a warming sun, living water, and soil filled with nutrients. I'm a landed immigrant, cared for and learning to accept the arborist's pruning, when needed. A little therapy, and a lot of laughter goes a long way, as I learn to love myself.

If she lacks wisdom, let her ask God, who gives it generously. Ask without doubting or be driven and tossed by the wind as a seed in flight. As she breathes His grace and mercy, she'll be spirit filled, her trunk strengthened, her heart filled, and her reaching limbs will speak from her soul gifting light. Belief, trust, and surrender enable her inner calm.

She is held and secure.

Living water constantly quenches her thirst and supports a growth of new branches, buds and leaves, and flowers that bloom and radiate joy. She knows His grace is sufficient and power is perfected in weakness.

When I am weak, then I am strong. I take a road less travelled, knowing I am complete in His presence.

I've been processing loss and journeying through grief for a lifetime. Recently, I learned of the significant relationship between love and loss. These are normal human experiences, and occasions we can prepare for, to be more adequately equipped to tend to grief. We will all grieve. If we love deeply, we grieve deeply. I've gained insight from the journey and today, June 2, 2021, I am ready.

Ready to let go, mourn, plant, and thrive.

~

It's just me here as I prepare to plant my tree. I want to plant her in our front yard, outside the living room window, where I will see it from our new recliner. "What do you think?"

I asked, then turned to read Dale's curiosity and the angle of his brow.

After I elaborated on my plan, Dale wholeheartedly agreed. After seasons of loss, without grace or skill to grieve tenderly, I've taken the time to process my grief and find an experienced counsellor. Someone who'll invest in the therapeutic relationship and earn my trust. It has taken years to advocate and access the supports I need. And then to trust and surrender to the work of healing.

Cornus nuttallii, also known as the Pacific dogwood, is native to western North America, and found in southwest British Columbia where I live, as well as in western Washington and Oregon and on the west slopes of the Californian mountain ranges. I was surprised to learn that the dogwoods' large white petals, the flowers I have loved since childhood, are called bracts. These showy white bracts form around a cluster of miniature, greenish flowers, called a flower-head.

An indigenous species, she thrives when each of five elements required for optimal growth are ensured. The Pacific dogwood was adopted in 1956 as British Columbia's floral emblem.

Species Mammalia, a.k.a. my Mamma, and her two infant saplings lived outside their native distributional range. A nurturer and deciduous flowering tree with camouflaged leaves and masks of many colours, Mom reforested, in the Comox Valley in the 1970s. One of her two grown seedlings has returned, come full circle, and is now rooted and maturing on the unceded territory of the Komox First Nation. Will she choose to listen, learn, and respect the Creator, the Earth, and its First Peoples with humility. Will she listen with an open heart and teachable spirit as her roots press outwards into a life-giving forest?

Mom moved beyond Calgary, Vancouver, Kamloops, and the Comox Valley, locations preferred by her species, both immediate and extended. A dogwood, her leaves were temperamental rather than robust, and did more than curl after a fire, and a season of storms which uprooted her marriage. The year 1966 would be an epic hurricane season for my mother, when her mother's life was cut short by cancer. Storms knocked her down, and left a jagged hole, a life without a husband or father for her children.

The final blow left Mom's roots raw and exposed, constantly in a state of shock, until dementia relieved her of her fears.

Tender hearted, impressionable saplings would grow and develop, imprinted by storms that impacted the parent like a chemical mark on a child's genes. Whether the weather directly or indirectly impacted our fragile roots, it affected our ability to thrive, in soil forever changed by human interactions.

My mother had travelled through the grassy and wooded areas where ticks feed, live, and roamed. She hadn't escaped when an unknown species questing lay in wait, then crawled onto my unsuspecting mother. Her fears and anxiety, like the tick, fastened itself to its host and burrowed deep. They burdened their host and her seeds' ability to send down tender roots as my mother moved and arrived in each new community.

Wherever she went, she dispersed mistrust like seeds, and an observant child listened and learned. When a dandelion turns to seed, as if by magic overnight, a delightful puffball appears. If only I could have closed my eyes and made a wish; I may have been able to stay.

I'd wished . . . someone would listen to my thoughts. Now, perhaps I was ready to take flight and, like a dandelion seed suspended from a parachute-like stalk, be released by a puff of breath and fly. My mind fluttered still, a dandelion seed alight on a gust of breeze.

~

With my supplies I prepared to dig. Dale offered to help; however, this was my project, my tree, and the closure

I required. There's a legend that suggested that it was a dogwood tree that provided the wood used to build the cross on which Jesus was crucified. The legend reminded me of God's promises, and each spring I knew I would look out my window with anticipation for those symbolic, white-petalled flowers I'd loved since I was a child.

# CHAPTER TWENTY-SIX

### I Dig

### (Take 2)

I was mindful of the journey that brought me here. Finally, I was ready to dig, be rooted and ready. Ready to answer questions: Who am I? Where do I belong?

Mamma lived through storms of emotion, masked and silenced, to protect us from what frightened her most. To escape fear, she moved to reorient and find stability. She housed herself on ocean currents, rather than docking with permanence in a safe harbour. Leaves on young saplings curled. Beyond daughter, my identity became: introduced immigrant, new girl at school, younger sister, second choice of new bedrooms, and uncertain of each new stomping ground on which I landed. In short, a girl seeking connection and longing to hear "I love you."

Seeking, I'd looked at my reflection in the lake and heard the awakening forest. Chickadees sang love songs and the brook babbled as it flowed coursing around embedded boulders. Evergreens emitted sweetness which lingered and filled my nostrils.

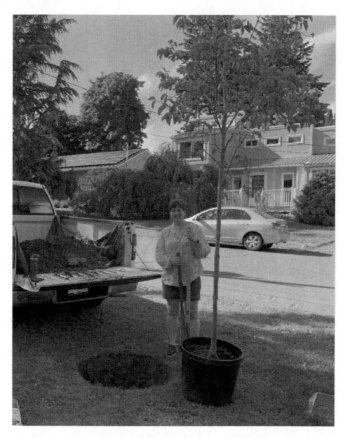

Pictured here with shovel and maddock, I'm ready. Dale takes my photo before heading off to give me space and time.

I'd tasted calm as I listened to the droplets on the window, my shoulders falling and jaw loosening, unclenched when I escaped into stories my imagination embellished. I sheltered beneath the mighty Douglas fir, who protected all below. Without affirmation, I'd known I could armour myself while I waited.

~

Dale left to run a few errands, after ensuring I had everything I required. Before leaving, he backed up the truck to the just right spot, readied the tarp in the back of the truck bed, and made sure the tailgate was down. He brought me both a shovel and mattock.

A mattock? Who knew what that was? Not I. Dale told me that a mattock, like a pickaxe, was used to break up the earth, especially when the ground is hard-packed and dry. We had very little precipitation in the summer of 2021. Under the sod of our front yard, embedded rocks might make digging a challenge.

Forever changed by love and the words of affection Dale lavished, we planted seeds. Two children would send down tender roots into healthy soil, interconnected in the web of family, faith, and community, secured by our unconditional love. When loved ones of the same species retired and drew closer, circling us with support, we thrived within an established, spectacular temperate rainforest and awe-inspiring ecosystem.

Slivers of wisdom, along with grey whispers, peek out along my hairline, and suggest lived experiences have woven their way into the fabric of my life. Through seasons of trauma, periods of overwhelming fear, loss and confusion, in addition to years of seeking, waiting, challenging myself to attain strength, while neglecting myself, I finally surrendered.

I trusted and believed I was worthy of care. I learned to appreciate the wisdom of grey; no longer finding a preference for black or white. Choosing to live in the bright, vibrant colours of language, paint, fabric, and ever-changing, growing relationships, which require care and hard work, I'm learning to love myself. Learning to listen and be alert to the feelings I experience, allowing myself to know the full range and not just the happy, positive, Pollyanna emotions.

I'm finding my thoughts interesting rather than absolute, and am seeking strategies which serve this unique, very rare normal, free-spirited, passionate human effectively. With my new GPS, a.k.a. roadmap, and emergency tool kit, a.k.a. my cell phone, I have choices to make, and am choosing to be proactive. I'm choosing to advocate for my health and wellness above the neck.

Highlights and colouring my hair to appear younger or masking the authentic me, getting stuck in anxious thoughts, listening to my Bossy Jocie (my inner critic), and using childish strategies, which no longer serve me, I leave these and more by the roadside.

Possibilities missed are mourned, and losses grieved. I've chosen to leave guilt and shame behind. It's time. Today is the perfect time to acknowledge, surrender, and outgrow what no longer serves my health and wellness.

Roots reach and sink deeper still. The right tree in the right place, connected in community and cared for; that's me.

Today, as I dig, I mourn and celebrate. I celebrate my career in gifted education, the students' lives I made a difference in, the important advocacy I rendered, and a career I loved. A career taken too soon, which left a festering wound. A wound which became infected like a virus spread throughout my body. Pain and response, which directly resulted from unresolved loss and grief.

Grief, like a tick, migrated to that warm, moist area of my body, found a desirable spot to draw blood and remain attached, wounding. Similarly, stressors found a receptive host lacking emotional resilience, previous wounds still raw and easily reopened, again by fresh intruders.

Without support or strategies, the tick found its way into my central nervous system and brain, where it caused neurological chaos. Its attack was met by a weakened, defenseless opposition of one, without armour or weapons. The brain, undefended, could no longer send and receive messages accurately.

I now live with FND, functional neurologic disorder. There is little known or even understood about this disorder. It has been under-researched for many years but is finally getting the attention it deserves. I am grateful, as researchers around the world are doing their best to find answers, and hopeful they will soon have better diagnostic protocols and treatment plans, in addition to a proactive strategy to educate more FND aware medical practitioners worldwide.

In addition, I live with other mental health diagnoses—OCD, PTSD and anxiety—although I am not defined by these either. I no longer suffer in silence. Instead, I speak up and out and I am fully aware of the need to advocate for oneself and prioritize self-care.

Prioritizing wellness is a daily choice for life.

~

I use the shovel to cut the sod around the circle where I've sprayed a ring of orange to mark the place, I've chosen to plant her, and then cut the sod into manageable chunks. Then I lift and remove the sod and begin to dig in earnest. Shortly thereafter, sweat trickles down my brow and face.

Dale arrives on scene with purpose, ready with another shovel in hand to help. He's always got my back.

"Step away, this is my project." Words I speak with such emphasis, I surprise myself, and Dale. He thoughtfully steps back in consideration of my expressed tone and body language. He's bilingual and speaks and understands both English and Jocelyn.

The pleaser interrupts and prepares to mask her truth: *I don't want your back, which is already in rough shape, to be in worse shape, or to exacerbate your already sore body.* But before this lie by omission even leaves my lips, I get the nudge to be honest and try again.

My not wanting help has nothing to do with Dale's sore back. It's about denial, loss, grief, pain and guilt, anger and bargaining, darkness, and physical decline. Mine.

It's about reconstruction and journeying through. It's about surrender, acceptance, growth, joy, and hope. Mine.

"I'm sorry," I say. "This is an important task for me alone. One heart, one shovel. It's me allowing myself to grieve, choosing to be tender with myself, and support my journey towards wellness. Thank you for your willingness to support me, Dale. I've got this."

Without comment and with lips sealed, and possibly a bleeding tongue, Dale smiles.

He gets me. Of this, I am certain. As he walks away, he leaves me with his trademark "Mmm," gets into his work truck and heads off. We've been married for thirty-eight years, and he knows me well.

In that moment, he deserves my heart and more, despite my hopelessness at deciphering the multitude of inflections and meanings of "Mmm."

I lean into my project and dig.

Quickly, I realize just how difficult this job will be despite my fierce determination. I stick with it, no matter the cost. I think of it as perseverance, an admirable quality. Family and friends call it stubbornness. The psychiatrist calls it OCD. Once I set a goal, it will be achieved.

Dale was not surprised by the OCD diagnosis, I'm sure. I've been lost to him for months since deciding to record my story. Writing with religious zeal, processing to understand the last seven years, and, well, *What the hell just happened?*

On my journey towards well-being, Dale gives me the prerequisite space, time, and love, even when he's lonely and goes without dinner .I'm lost in my writing and oblivious to the passage of time. He's willing to wait. He'd reassured me afterwards, saying, "I'm delighted to see you smile again." And "I'm so proud of you, Jocelyn."

My neighbor from across the street asks in a serious tone, "Do you have a permit to dig?"

My anxiety skyrockets. I don't. But then I look up and realize he's grinning; his aim was to get a rise out of me. It worked. Gullible may as well be my middle name. Keith, just like the neighbour, loves pushing my buttons, pulling levers, and figuring out how things work, always has, always will.

"It's just too much fun not to push your buttons, Mom," he'll say with a smirk.

While Dale's gone, I continue to dig. Sweat now pours down my brow and dampens my shirt. I'm making extremely slow progress. Then, in a flash of much-needed insight, I remember. There's a tool Dale offered, explained, and showed me how to use: a mattock. It's beside the lawn chair, which he brought as a gentle reminder and encouragement to take breaks. He knows when I'm laser focused; I forget to stay hydrated and release the throttle. My usual tempo, full speed.

Unaware that Dale had long since returned home, and in the zone, I point the shovel, step up on the back metal digging part, where the handle meets metal, and use my weight to lean in and dig. And repeat.

Stepping back, occasionally, I remind myself, *Bend your knees; it'll save your back.* Then I return to bending, reaching, lifting, and turning to dump the soil into the back of the pickup truck bed, where Dale placed a tarp, to make unloading and cleanup simplified.

I stop occasionally for sips, and to wipe sweat from my eyes, but the plastic water bottle, sitting so long in the blistering sun, no longer refreshes. The ice has long since melted.

The hole takes shape but looks like an inverted ice cream cone. The sides are slanted, and hard packed with embedded boulders. Reaching for the mattock, I attempt to lift it using one hand. Whoa, it's heavy. I try again with two. Grasping and lifting it again, I attempt to use it as Dale demonstrated. Dale is much stronger, though, and as I bring it down into the hole, I'm grateful for a near miss. I almost lop of my left foot.

A picture instantly reappears from the deep recesses of my mind. I'm in my early twenties, with an axe, and remember an unsuccessful attempt to chop kindling. I can still feel the rush of adrenaline and the thud of the descending axe. A knife in soft butter had chopped right through my running shoe between my big toe and the little piggie that stayed home. I'd been thankful to still have five.

I widen my stance proactively and swing the mattock again. Sweat now streams into my eyes, stinging painfully. However, I am successful. I break loose enough dirt around a football size boulder near the base of the hole. With effort, I pull it from the rock-shaped cavity. A smile escapes. When I attempt to lift the rock out, I'm suddenly aware of the height from the base of the hole to the tailgate. And boy oh boy, that sucker's heavy.

I newly appreciate labourers and ditch diggers who do this repetitive work, and I feel embarrassed that I've been proud of such a minor accomplishment. I'm needy and dependent on the strength of others and blessed to have people in my life who will support me with their strengths when I ask.

Looking over at my tree awaiting transplant, I see I still have another foot of dirt and rock to excavate to make room for the root ball. I don't complain, slow, or take breaks. This is my work, my healing, my choice, and I take ownership and responsibility for each decision.

I alternate between shovel and mattock until my endeavor is complete and then slump into the lawn chair, remembering another chair.

One I fell into happily exhausted, on a Friday, in May 2014, and then again, in February 2021, when I experienced central apnea, and seized.

With gratitude, on June 4, 2021, I am physically well enough to manage this digging. I'm grateful for the miracle I've been gifted of restored physical, emotional, and spiritual strength, and support from many, all of whom have enabled me to journey towards mental health and wellness. I pause and reflect with gratitude.

The hole, I judge, is ready. I look up to where there is now a huge mound of dirt, sod, and rock lifted one shovel at a time into the back of the pickup truck and am not surprised that, like after a marathon seizure, I'm spent.

It's time. Tension cries from taut, strained muscles and my back is tender from repetitive lifting as I kneel. I appreciate being alone. My face and arms are covered with dirt, sweat, and the scent of labour. I'm bone tired, and as I reach out, I'm relaxed and at peace. I've chosen to bury an artifact, the last copy of a letter, which triggered such painful grief. A copy of the email I'd written, as well as a copy of the Letter of Direction which was placed on my personnel file after the disciplinary meeting in 2014. Selected to symbolize love, loss, and grief.

I have loved, and I have grieved. My truth has been acknowledged. I've gained insight and chosen to listen with a teachable spirit. I'm learning to process my lived experiences and to choose a healing path to journey through seasons of love, loss, and grief. With gratitude, I choose to let go of outdated beliefs about grief and to nurture and support my grief with tenderness and love. I choose to re-humanize grief and to live a life changed by loss, knowing I'm loved.

I reach to where the letters lie folded on the other side of the hole. Glancing briefly at them, not giving either more attention than needed, I take the lighter and flick the switch.

They're afire. I'm mesmerized as I observe the slow burn. Hypnotized, I kneel in stillness. I close my eyes and am beside the ocean listening to the sounds of the waves gently washing up against the shore, with the moon casting blessings against the night sky. It's poetic. Creation calls.

I exhale and find a sense of calm as ash descends. Gently, gliding like a gull on the wind currents before diving. Ash falls on the fresh-scented earth. With humility, I reach and collect a handful of soil. Tenderly, I sprinkle earth atop ash, caressing a baby's bottom and hear a whisper, *I love you.*

With caution, I remove the canvas, which held her root ball securely. I, too, have longed to be held. She is extremely vulnerable, exposed in this way. There's only a brief barrier of clay shielding her roots. Unlike her thin shield, I'm at last armoured and protected in choosing to surrender and trust.

I've prepared her, know her, and am ready to love fully. In surrender, I listen, acknowledge grief, and have learned it's okay that I'm not okay. I've done what I needed to do. Alone.

I knew. She'd known, but feared she'd be judged and abandoned. She's learning to reach and branch out to share her story. I know now she'd needed help. She needed and was worthy of the supports she required, so I advocate and acquire the care she deserves because I love her.

I'm mentally prepared to lower the dogwood into the hole. How can I be sure the root ball in its state of fragility isn't damaged? I've been there. I've been her, in this fragile state, needing pencil poles and prayers to tether and support me.

Dale knowingly waited. Now ready, I ask, and he agrees to help. One hand under another, together, supporting her and each other, we bend our knees simultaneously to protect aging, weary bodies, his and mine.

Mine from jerking, seizing, and now digging, his from an injury in his teens, and a lifetime of hard work. He's always got my back. Together, as we had on our first date in 1982, we share the load. And, together, we lower this indigenous beauty into the earth, where she belongs. Tenderly, prepared for transplant, now with rebounding joy, mourning is over. I add water, bone meal, fertilizer, fresh new soil, and exhale a promise of welcome and invitation to grow deep roots. Mine, hers, and ours.

Together, Dale and I pat down the cool, damp soil, adding layer upon layer, two shovels at a time until there's no longer a grave. Fear isn't in the driver's seat any longer. Unless, of course, along the way, I accidentally take a wrong exit off the freeway. And I will. I'm human.

Instead, I look out the window at a vibrant young tree, a celebration of my life and love. I choose to speak about the reality of love and loss, as well as the connection between loving deeply and grieving deeply. I want to become skilled at grieving and in supporting others in their grief; because if we love, we will grieve. It's just a matter of time.

With soil between my fingers and a sense of a new connection with the earth, I exhale. Calm infiltrates each neuron and every fiber of my being. With knowledge and a belief in the interconnectedness of all living things, the web of life, the parts, which make me whole, I know now she'll be nourished for years to come. She's thirsty for living water, as am I.

JOCELYN BYSTROM

# EPILOGUE

Dearest Jocelyn,

Your story starts when you choose to start sharing it and stops when you're finished telling it. Yours is a true story; and of course, this is not the end.

I love you, Jocelyn.

Life, like a blessing, is not something that you can imagine. Neither, where it will go, or how it will end. It promises of course never to go in a straight line. Know with certainty, beloved one, that you don't sit, stand, or kneel alone.

You are loved.

I admire your creativity, your courage and tenacity, and your strong visceral connection with the natural world. Breathe freely.

I appreciate your teachable spirit and the bravery to risk: being alone, making mistakes, failure, and rejection. Risk coupled with trust revitalizes connection. You've grown. You've learned, you've reflected and are coming into your fullness. I've noticed.

I value that you've given voice to a story that's yours alone. It begged to be told. May the seeds you've planted nourish hungry hearts, like yours.

I've witnessed a heart opening, walls tumbling, and a voice asserting itself. May this enable you to express your deep appreciation for life, trust that you are not alone, and that I am God.

You stood, you stand, and wonder. You stare into the glass and ask: *Am I enough?*

Look instead beyond your thoughts and see the facts. You are in bloom.

Love Always,
That Girl You Consider in Reflection.

# REFERENCES

*About – (FND)*. (n.d.). Functional Neurological Disorder (FND) – A Patient's Guide to FND. https://neurosymptoms.org/en/about/

*Assertiveness*. (2019, 10). CCI - Anxiety, Depression, Bipolar and Eating Disorders - Perth. https://www.cci.health.wa.gov.au/Resources/Looking-After-Yourself/Assertiveness

Corrigan, P. W., and Rao, D. (2012). On the self-stigma of mental illness: Stages, disclosure, and strategies for change. *The Canadian Journal of Psychiatry, 57*(8), 464-469. https://doi.org/10.1177/070674371205700804

Devine, M. (2017). *It's OK that you're not OK: Meeting grief and loss in a culture that doesn't understand*. Sounds True.

Everett, L. (2021, April 6). Looking beyond the critical challenges: Self-care is a key part of the mental health conversation. *The ATA NEWS*, p. 11.

(2023, May 11). FND Hope International. https://fndhope.org/

Ganssle, G. (2022, March 3). *The lent project*. Biola University Center for Christianity, Culture and the

Arts. https://ccca.biola.edu/lent/2022/#day-mar-10

Huang, L. (2022, April 10). *The lent project.* Biola University Center for Christianity, Culture and the Arts. https://ccca.biola.edu/lent/2022/#day-apr-10

Kaculini, C. M., Tate-Looney, A. J., and Seifi, A. (2021, March 17). *The history of epilepsy: From ancient mystery to modern misconception.* https://doi.org/10.7759/cureus.13953

Kolk, B. A. (2015). *The body keeps the score: Brain, mind, and body in the healing of trauma.* Penguin Books.

Levine, P. A., and Kline, M. (2010). *Trauma through a child's eyes: Awakening the ordinary miracle of healing.* North Atlantic Books.

Maté, G. (2011). *When the body says no: The cost of hidden stress.* Vintage Canada.

Maté, G. (2022). *The myth of normal: Trauma, illness, and healing in a toxic culture.* Knopf Canada.

May, R. (2009). *Man's search for himself.* W. W. Norton & Company.

National Alliance on Mental Illness. (2020). *The ripple effect of mental illness.* NAMI: National Alliance on Mental Illness. https://www.nami.org/NAMI/media/NAMI-Media/Infographics/NAMI_Impact_RippleEffect_2020_FINAL.pdf

National Alliance on Mental Illness. (2022). *NAMI: National Alliance on Mental Illness.* NAMI: National Alliance on Mental Illness. Retrieved April 23, 2022, from https://www.nami.org/NAMI/media/NAMI-Media/Infographics/NAMI_2020MH_ByTheNumbers_Youth-r.pdf

Scamvougeras, A., and Howard, A. (2018). *Understanding and managing somatoform disorders: A guide for clinicians.*

Schuster, D. (2022, March 21). *The lent project.* Biola University Center for Christianity, Culture and the Arts. https://ccca.biola.edu/lent/2022/#day-mar-21

Stone, J. (2009). *Functional neurological disorder (FND) – A patient's guide to FND*. Functional Neurological Disorder (FND) – A Patient's Guide to FND. https://neurosymptoms.org/en/

Wagner, D. (2016, June 27). *Polyvagal theory in practice.* Counseling Today: A Publication of the American Counseling Association. Retrieved May 13, 2022, from https://ct.counseling.org/2016/06/polyvagal-theory-practice/

Walker, P. (2013). *Complex PTSD : From surviving to thriving: A guide and map for recovering from childhood trauma.* Createspace Independent Publishing Platform.

Wang, M. (2021, February 19). *The lent project.* Biola University Center for Christianity, Culture and the Arts. https://ccca.biola.edu/lent/2021/#day-feb-19

*What is FND*. (2023, June 27). FND Hope International. https://fndhope.org/fnd-guide/

# ACKNOWLEDGEMENT

I would like to acknowledge that I live, work, learn and worship on the traditional territories of the K'ómoks First Nation. I would like to thank them for the privilege of living on their land. I acknowledge the K'ómoks people, as the Care takers of the "land of plenty" since time immemorial.

FiNDing Hope began to take shape as I journaled medical distress and medication trials as my cognition declined, and I hadn't known why. Over time, the writing shifted to writing through a lens of gratitude, and as a therapeutic and creative outlet, as I struggled. I'd needed to discharge the tough stuff, that I couldn't voice aloud. I am grateful for the extraordinary circle of grace that has encompassed me as I worked on this book, as well as those at the very top of my gratitude list: my beloved husband, Dale, and our adult children, Keith Bystrom and Kristen Basaraba, as well as Kristen's husband Matthew Basaraba.

I am blessed and grateful for my dear friends: Sharon, Rosanne, Mary, Heather, Cindy, Rory, Pippa, Teri, Billie, Ken, and Jill. Each of these beautiful humans lifted me when I was overwhelmed by the complexity of my physical and mental health deterioration.

Confidentiality is a sacred tenet every educator, school counsellor, and each of my dear friend's holds dear. Many individuals in this story consented to the sharing of their identities and our shared stories without altering any details that would provide them anonymity. Their real names are used with permission. Other names, of medical professionals, colleagues, employers, and hundreds of students, are representative of individuals that I've had the honour and privilege to work and learn alongside throughout my twenty-five-plus years as an educator.

For my colleagues through the years, you've taught me that teaching isn't a job for one person alone, and I'm sincerely grateful. It takes a community of care, and each of you continue to provide inspiration, encouragement and proverbial sunshine. In 1986, as a brand new university graduate, and very green teaching credentials I naively believed, I could change everything. That my passion and hard work would be enough. I know better now. I've needed you. Thank you.

We're stronger together, as we come alongside each other with curiosity and kindness. You've taught me teach with humility, a teachable spirit, and a growth mindset.

For the many incredible medical practitioners I've crossed paths with seeking care. Thank you! I'm exceptionally grateful to: Dr(s). JJ. Sidhu, J. Percy, J. Tham, S. Cresswell, R. Carruthers, J. Valerio, J. Barton, C. Hrazdil, S. Yip, J. Tan, N. Hope, and S. Olsen, and the incredible team at Westward Medical, in the Comox Valley. You listened, saw me, heard me and are exemplars of what every individual wants and needs from their medical care providers. My life mattered, you cared. I'm immeasurably indebted to each of you for my joy-filled life in 2023.

Your collaborative trauma-informed care helped me to thrive, grow, and heal as I learned to prioritize self-compassion and care. I've learned to assert myself, advocate for my health and well-being, and I'm prayerful that each of you will mindfully prioritize your own health and wellness, relationships, family, and values, especially as you find yourselves working overtime, and long hours caring for your patients. Thank you. Your support mattered.

I observed the long hours, appreciated the supportive phone calls made after hours and on the Eve, of your Christmas holidays, Dr. Percy. To the crew at Vancouver General, Seizures Investigative Unit SIU: Thank you. You worked diligently with an exceptional level of professionalism during the global pandemic to ensure patients like me were well cared for, with compassion, despite difficult working conditions in 2021. Thank you for digging deep for answers, information and a diagnosis that made sense. I was blessed to be referred to compassionate medical practitioners with masterful expertise at a time when I struggled with confusion and uncertainty. Thank you for persisting when my hands and mind were rigid and claw-like, and as astonished eyes & amygdala grappled to comprehend, an unexpected FND diagnosis. Thank you, for signing on the dotted line, for referrals, and triple checking all the boxes to ensure I knew I could count on respectful, collaborative, and continuing care.

The list of people who made it possible for this book to come into the light, and out of the darkness that filled my mind, is almost as long as the numbered pages in FiNDing Hope. Please know that each of you made a difference. This acknowledgement is for you! I'm grateful beyond what you can imagine. You had my back, and your prayers lifted me when it mattered most. Forgive my lack of named acknowledgements face to face. I'm forever grateful. You know who you are.

I'm sincerely grateful for friends who offered rides to the North East Woods for soul-quenching early morning walks. Being able to enjoy the love and light filtering through the canopy as Ollie, my mental health fur buddy, and I skipped over rocks and roots and listened to the awakening forest and chirping birds meant everything to me. Always, the northwest breezes promised our favourite kind weather. Hopeful.

To the many writing mentors, who came alongside me with wisdom and willingness.

Thank you. Your shared gifts and knowledge were offered with lavish generosity. Without your kindness and encouragement, I wouldn't have had the courage to speak up, record my life blunders, or overcome my anxiety on the steep learning curve to becoming a published author. Each of you created brave spaces for me to practice, fail, and eventually thrive as a new writer. I want to thank Rebecca Gifford, William (Bill) Israel, Meghan Flaherty, Sally Dean, Nicole Severance, Hannah Wiseheart, Natalie Goldberg, Patrick Guindon, and my fellow 'shoppers: Jeremy Goldstein, Aliah Wright, Walter Pryor, and Jaye Landon, who came alongside me every Wednesday for nearly a year gifting me with generous critiques, feedback and encouragement.

For Jeff Ourvan, my writing coach and publisher, I am filled with deepest gratitude. Your invitation to participate with a gifted group of serious writers enabled me to believe I that I could be a real writer too. You became a trusted ally, confidant, coach, and undisputable champion, as I learned to share my story, and complete the labor of love that has become *FiNDing Hope*. You made it easy trust you Jeff! And, you know me well. I don't trust easily. You have been a true partner in this passion project from Day One, and I'm grateful for your belief in me from the start. For weekly feedback, for developmental editing, and so much more. Thank you!

For Patrick Price, my editor, I owe immeasurable gratitude. You believed in my writing and replied to my bold request to critique my first three chapters and blew me away when you said that I was a stronger writer than I believed. For your offer to mentor me with coaching calls as I got started, and your "yes" to a final full edit. Thank you! I knew from the start, despite my being in Comox, British Columbia, and Canadian, and that you lived in New York, USA, that you cared about my story. Each time you provided editorial input, you provided me with so much more than editing. You gifted me a rare source of sustenance, strength, and learning. And oh boy, did I have a lot to learn. Patrick, your editorial genius gifted me and went way beyond expectations for proofreading and finishing touches. I'm sincerely grateful for the love and finesse you brought to my story, as I dreamt to share it with the literary world, mental health and FND (Functional Neurologic Disorder) communities. I'm honoured to have worked alongside you.

For my mother, Sydney Carole Hall,
You loved us immeasurably, even without words, and gave up much so that we could have the world. It was an absolute honour to come alongside you as care partner, after the years of generosity, and parenting you shouldered. Even as your life took an unexpected zag with a diagnosis of frontal temporal dementia you humbly continued to teach me to love God, use my gifts in service, and come alongside others with kindness and curiosity. You've modelled unconditional love through your actions and faith, and unquestionable resilience in the face of adversity. You taught me to believe in myself, and I'll long remember that you believed in me. It's impossible to do justice here to the endless sacrifices you made for us, for your grandchildren, and for our family. May you rest peacefully in the gentle arms of Jesus, free from the cares and challenges of this world. I'm grateful for your life, your love, and your presence in mine knowing that you're smiling down from heaven. I've finally succumbed to the deliciousness of eggs and toast, Mom. And Dale and I can't eat vanilla ice cream without smiling. As I kneel to pray in church, you are there. As I walk at the Filberg Park, you are present there too. So very many precious moments we've shared. I love you, Mom.

For Keith, our first born.
Thank you! For your love and loyalty . . . and presence; whenever I've needed you most, you show up without being

asked. For pushing my buttons, most of the time, and knowing when not to . Thank you. For your delicious wit, and sense of humor. You bless me and I adore having a good belly laugh with you. I love you, despite your telling me that you won't read my book unless I buy you a copy. Just wait and hold your breath, maybe there'll be one waiting for you in your Christmas stocking. Though possibly your curiosity will make you pay the price sooner. Time will tell.

For Kristen, our precious daughter.
Your actions speak volumes. Your prayers and presence have held me when I feared. I only hope that I can repay you with the unconditional love, you've so freely given. Thank you for the gifts of your time, your patience, and presence at so many medical appointments, as well as in the making of precious memories. I love you.

For my beloved husband, Dale,
You chose me, prioritized me, and have loved me since our first date in August 1982. Thank you for daily reminders that I'm beautiful. There are no words to express the extent of my gratitude! You're my guy, my handsome Swede, and my best friend. My love for you has no limits. I have certainly put the vows you made to me to the test. Through sickness and in health, our love has stood the test of time. You have my heart, and always have. Thank you, for the many nights you lay in bed and wondered where your wife was as I wrote way past the witching hour. Thank you. Your words of affection bless me. Knowing that you're proud of me, fills me. I firmly believe that you've got my back. You rocked in your role as seizure partner, even when it wasn't a role you wanted. Who could have imagined as you stared with adoration into my nineteen year old eyes at twenty-one, that's what you meant when you promised , I do!

Thank you for never leaving me as I experienced unspeakable fear during seizures. The love you gift me with daily is rock solid, and I'm blessed to be in love with my best friend. I'm here for you, too. Take good care of the man I adore.

# ABOUT THE AUTHOR

## Jocelyn Bystrom

Jocelyn completed an M.Ed. in Educational Leadership & Counselling from City University of Seattle. She's an educator and writer who has made a name for herself in British Columbia as an educational leader, K-8th grade 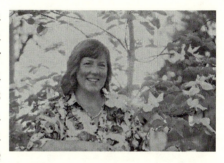 teacher, Adlerian School Counsellor, and Gifted Education Specialist. Jocelyn Bystrom is a self-described articulate, career-minded perfectionist. She has a special passion for mental health advocacy and works alongside mental health leaders & stigma-free advocates to eliminate the stigma surrounding mental health in her Western Canada community, in schools, in the workplace and online. Jocelyn blogs to share mental health and FND health content at www.FNDingHope.com with the aim of sharing mental health insights, resources, and wisdom. She also has several thousand social media followers across Twitter, Instagram, and Facebook.

Made in the USA
Middletown, DE
09 August 2024

58835257R00217